MALIGNANCY AND THE HEMOSTATIC SYSTEM

MONOGRAPHS OF
THE MARIO NEGRI INSTITUTE FOR
PHARMACOLOGICAL RESEARCH, MILAN

Series Editor: Silvio Garattini

Amphetamines and Related Compounds
Edited by E. Costa and S. Garattini, 1970, 976 pp.

Basic and Therapeutic Aspects of Perinatal Pharmacology
Edited by P. L. Morselli, S. Garattini, and F. Sereni, 1975, 456 pp.

The Benzodiazepines
Edited by S. Garattini, E. Mussini, and L. O. Randall, 1973, 707 pp.

Central Mechanisms of Anorectic Drugs
Edited by S. Garattini and R. Samanin, 1978, 502 pp.

Chemotherapy of Cancer Dissemination and Metastasis
Edited by S. Garattini and G. Franchi, 1973, 400 pp.

Drug Interactions
Edited by P. L. Morselli, S. Garattini, and S. N. Cohen, 1974, 416 pp.

Factors Affecting the Action of Narcotics
Edited by M. W. Adler, L. Manara, and R. Samanin, 1978, 787 pp.

Frontiers in Therapeutic Drug Monitoring
Edited by G. Tognoni, R. Latini, and W. J. Juska, 1980, 188 pp.

Glutamic Acid: Advances in Biochemistry and Physiology
*Edited by L. J. Filer, Jr., S. Garattini, M. R. Kare, W. A. Reynolds, and
R. J. Wurtman, 1979, 416 pp.*

Hemostatsis, Prostaglandins, and Renal Diseases
Edited by G. Remuzzi, G. Mecca, and G. de Gaetano, 1980, 460 pp.

Insolubilized Enzymes
Edited by Salmona, C. Saronio, and S. Garattini, 1974, 236 pp.

Interactions Between Putative Neurotransmitters in the Brain
Edited by S. Garattini, J. F. Pujol, and R. Samanin, 1978, 380 pp.

Isolated Liver Perfusion and Its Applications
Edited by I. Bartošek, A. Guaitani, and L. L. Miller, 1973, 303 pp.

Mass Spectrometry in Biochemistry and Medicine
Edited by A. Frigerio and N. Castagnoli, Jr., 1974, 379 pp.

Pharmacology of Steroid Contraceptive Drugs
Edited by S. Garattini and H. W. Berendes, 1977, 391 pp.

Platelets: A Multidisciplinary Approach
Edited by G. de Gaetano and S. Garattini, 1978, 500 pp.

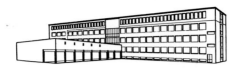

MONOGRAPHS OF
THE MARIO NEGRI INSTITUTE FOR
PHARMACOLOGICAL RESEARCH, MILAN

Malignancy and the Hemostatic System

Edited by

Maria Benedetta Donati, M.D.
*Head, Laboratory for Haemostatsis
and Thrombosis Research
Istituto di Ricerche Farmacologiche
"Mario Negri"
Milan, Italy*

John F. Davidson, M.D.
*Consultant Haematologist
Royal Infirmary
Glasgow, United Kingdom*

Silvio Garattini, M.D.
*Director, Istituto di Ricerche Farmacologiche
"Mario Negri"
Milan, Italy*

Raven Press ■ New York

Raven Press, 1140 Avenue of the Americas, New York, New York 10036

Made in the United States of America

Great care has been taken to maintain the accuracy of the information contained in the volume. However, Raven Press cannot be held responsible for errors or for any consequences arising from the use of the information contained herein.

Library of Congress Cataloging in Publication Data

Main entry under title:

Malignancy and the hemostatic system.

    (Monographs of the Mario Negri Institute for Pharmacological Research, Milan)
    Includes bibliographical references and index.
    1. Metastasis. 2. Hemostasis. 3. Cancer –
Complications and sequelae. I. Donati, Maria
Benedetta. II. Davidson, John Forsyth.
III. Garattini, Silvio. IV. Series: Istituto
di ricerche farmacologiche Mario Negri. Monographs.

[DNLM: 1. Neoplasms – Complications. 2. Hemo-
stasis. QZ 200 M2486]
   RC269. M34   616.99'407   80-39949
ISBN 0-89004-463-5

Preface

It is the aim of this volume to present an updated state of the art concerning the complex interactions between the hemostatic system and the biology of tumor growth and metastasis.

The existence of such interactions has long been suspected, but their specific pathogenic and clinical implications still await definition. Reviewed herein are the various mechanisms whereby cancer cells may interact with the hemostatic system; these are the role of cancer cell–endothelium interplay in metastasis formation, the ability of cancer cells to induce platelet aggregation, and the pathways of activation of coagulation and/or fibrinolysis by malignant cells.

In addition, experimental models used thus far for the study of *in vivo* fibrin–cancer cell interactions are critically examined. Finally, the clinical relevance of anticoagulation in the treatment of cancer is discussed.

Cell biologists and hematologists should find that this volume, with its contributions from a continually developing field, will provide the stimulus for a multidisciplinary approach to the biology of tumor cell dissemination and of cellular hemostasis.

Maria Benedetta Donati
John F. Davidson
Silvio Garattini

Contents

1 Malignancy and Hemostasis: Introduction
  G. V. R. Born

5 Cancer Cell–Endothelial Reactions: The Microinjury Hypothesis
  and Localized Thrombosis in the Formation of
  Micrometastases
  B. A. Warren

27 *In Vitro* Mechanism of Platelet Aggregation by Purified Plasma
   Membrane Vesicles Shed by Mouse 15091A Tumor Cells
   *Gabriel J. Gasic, James L. Catalfamo, Tatiana B. Gasic,
   and Nebojsa Avdalovic*

37 The *In Vitro* Activity of Platelet Aggregating Material from
   SV-40 Transformed Mouse 3T3 Fibroblasts
   Simon Karpatkin and Edward Pearlstein

57 Cancer Cell Procoagulant Activity
   H. R. Gralnick

65 Pathways of Blood Clotting Initiation by Cancer Cells
   N. Semeraro and M. B. Donati

83 Plasminogen Activator Released from Malignant
   Ovarian Tumors
   B. Astedt

89 Fibrin and Cancer Cell Growth: Problems in the
   Evaluation of Experimental Models
   Anreina Poggi, Maria Benedetta Donati, and Silvio Garattini

103 The Use of Oral Anticoagulants in Tumor Therapy
    P. Hilgard

113 Anticoagulation in the Treatment of Cancer in Man
    Leo R. Zacharski

129 Haemostasis and Malignancy
    J. F. Davidson and I. D. Walker

133 *Subject Index*

Contributors

B. Astedt
*Departments of Gynecology and
   Obstetrics in Malmo and Lund
University of Lund
S-22185 Lund, Sweden*

Nebosja Avdalovic
*Wistar Institute
Philadelphia, Pennsylvania 19104*

G. V. R. Born
*Pharmacology Department
King's College
University of London
London, United Kingdom*

James L. Catalfamo
*Department of Pathology
University of Pennsylvania
School of Medicine
Philadelphia, Pennsylvania 19104*

J. F. Davidson
*Department of Haematology
Royal Infirmary
Glasgow, United Kingdom*

M. B. Donati
*Istituto di Ricerche Farmacologiche
   "Mario Negri"
20157 Milan, Italy*

Silvio Garattini
*Istituto di Ricerche Farmacologiche
   "Mario Negri"
20157 Milan, Italy*

Gabriel J. Gasic
*Department of Pathology
University of Pennsylvania
School of Medicine
Philadelphia, Pennsylvania 19104*

Tatiana B. Gasic
*Department of Pathology
University of Pennsylvania
School of Medicine
Philadelphia, Pennsylvania 19104*

H. R. Gralnik
*Hematology Service
Clinical Pathology Department
Clinical Center
National Institutes of Health
Bethesda, Maryland 20205*

P. Hilgard
*Department of Haematology
Royal Postgraduate Medical School
Hammersmith Hospital
London W12 OHS, United Kingdom*

Simon Karpatkin
*The Departments of Medicine and
   Pathology
   and Irvington House Institute
New York University, Medical School
New York, New York 10016*

Edward Pearlstein
*The Departments of Medicine and
   Pathology
   and Irvington House Institute
New York University Medical School
New York, New York 10016*

Andreina Poggi
*Istituto di Ricerche Farmacologiche
   "Mario Negri"
20157 Milan, Italy*

N. Semeraro
*Istituto di Ricerche Farmacologiche
   "Mario Negri"
20157 Milan, Italy;
and Department of Microbiology,
University of Bari, Bari, Italy*

I. D. Walker
*Department of Haematology
Royal Infirmary
Glasgow, United Kingdom*

B. A. Warren
Department of Pathology
University of Western Ontario
London, Ontario, Canada

Leo R. Zacharski
Dartmouth Medical School
Veterans Administration Hospital
White River Junction, Vermont 05001

Malignancy and the Hemostatic System,
edited by M. B. Donati et al.
Raven Press, New York © 1981.

Malignancy and Hemostasis: Introduction

G. V. R. Born

Pharmacology Department, King's College
University of London, London, United Kingdom

Processes of malignancy and of haemostasis can in principal interact in both directions: that is, malignant growths could affect haemostasis and components involved in haemostasis could affect malignant growths.

Interactions in the first direction are exemplified by the association of subacute defibrination with disseminated malignant diseases (Marder, Weiner, Shulman & Shapiro, 1949; Merskey, Johnson, Kleiner & Woho, 1967). Such defibrinations have been described in association with cancers at breast, lung, prostate, stomach, colon, pancreas or gall bladder, although only rarely with the various leukaemias or Hodgkins disease.

Interactions in the other direction have come under increasing scrutiny recently, particularly as part of investigations into metastasis. Hints were repeatedly picked up that the successful metastasizing of tumor cells was influenced crucially by fibrin and platelets. The magnitude of these efforts has two important reasons: first, observations on the fundamental change in malignancy (Harris, 1971) give little hope of our ever being able to prevent initiation of the disease. This work indicates the operation of two essential processes: generation of genetic variation in a cell population as a whole, and selection by the body of certain specific variants that are capable of progressive growth. If these conclusions should hold for human malignancies, a tumour-inducing agent need not be highly specific in the genetic lesions that it induces. It would be enough if such an agent increased genetic variation in the exposed cell population to a point where the specific lesions responsible for malignancy, although random events, had a high probability of occurring. Tumour inducing agents such as chemical carcinogens, radiation or even oncogenic viruses would then act, not by converting normal to malignant cells, but by generating enough genetic variation to permit malignant variants to occur with predictable frequency.

Such a probabilistic interpretation of malignancy implies that the vast majority of the variants produced, and hence the vast majority of chromosomal aberrations, are irrelevant to the production of the malignant state. On the other hand, another implication is that there always remains a finite probability of the production of the chromosomal lesion responsible for malignancy, because it is inconceivable that every type of oncogenic agent could be eliminated from the external and internal environment. Moreover, it would seem to be impossible to anticipate which cell or cells out of the exceedingly large number of cells making up the body will suffer the particular chromosomal lesion responsible for malignant change.

On the other hand, metastatic spreading of malignant growths is likely to depend on various physiological factors which it may indeed be possible to modify therapeutically. This would apply particularly to haemostatic mechanisms, so that the demonstration of such dependence could well indicate new ways of preventing secondary growth which are, after all, most commonly responsible for the patients' disablement and death.

It is known that when malignant cells are injected experimentally into the circulation, the vast majority rapidly become nonviable. In endogenous malignant diseases the entry of cells into the circulation is presumably continuous, become detached from the primary tumour intermittently as single cells or as small clumps. How this difference affects the variability of the cells in the blood stream is not certain. However, it is reasonable to presume that only small proportions of such endogenous cells survive as potential progenators of metastasis. An all-important question is, therefore, whether any components of the haemostatic process favour the survival and implantation of circulating malignant cells. For example, does an association of circulating tumour cells with the platelets favour adhesion to vascular endothelium (Warren, 1978; Gasic et al., 1978; Ambrus et al., 1978)?

These problems and many others were considered as thoroughly and critically as the evidence permitted at a Symposium on Malignancy and Haemostasis held during the VIIth International Congress on Thrombosis and Haemostasis, July 1979. The Chairman, Dr. Benedetta Donati, and her contributors are to be commended for their efforts to bring together what knowledge we have so far. That they also reveal the gaps in this knowledge will serve to spur further research into an aspect of malignancy which is so important clinically.

Just to widen our thinking about connections between malignant disease and the blood vascular system, it may be worth recalling that tumour cells apparently produce an agent capable of inducing the growth of blood vessels. This "tumor angiogenesis factor" confers on malignant tumours the ability to stimulate proliferation of new capillaries and thereby appears to be essential for progressive tumour growth (Folkman, 1974). It is intriguing to wonder whether the vessels induced by this factor are wholly like vessels elsewhere, or whether the haemorrhagic tendency in tumours derives, at least in part, from some peculiarities of intra-tumour vessels. On the other hand, another explanation could be that the malignant environment somehow diminishes the effectiveness of local haemostatic processes. This indicates the relevance of this question to this Symposium.

REFERENCES

Ambrus, J.L., Ambrus, C.M. and Gastpar, H. (1978): Studies on platelet aggregation and platelet interaction with tumor cells. In: Platelets: a multidisciplinary approach. G. de Gaetano and S. Garattini (eds.) Raven Press: New York, 467-480.

Folkman, J. (1974): Tumour angiogenesis factor. Cancer Research, 34, 2109-2113.

Gasic, G.J., Boettiger, D., Catalfamo, J.L., Gasic, T.B. and Stewart, G.J. (1978): Platelet interactions in malignancy and cell transformation: functional and biochemical studies. In: Platelets: a multidisciplinary approach. G. de Gaetano and S. Garattini (eds.) Raven Press: New York, 447-456.

Harris, H. (1971): Cell fusion and the analysis of malignancy. Proc.Royal Soc.B., 179, 1-8.

Marder, M., Weiner, M., Shulman, P. and Shapiro, S. (1949): Afibrinogenaemia occurring in the case of malignancy of the prostate with bone metastasis. N.Y.State J.Med., 49, 1197-1203

Merskey, J., Johnson, A.J., Kleiner, G.J. and Woho, H. (1967): The defibrination syndrome; clinical features and laboratory diagnosis. Br.J.Haematol. 13, 528-531

Warren, B.A. (1978): Platelet-tumour cell interactions: morphological studies. In: Platelets: a multidisciplinary approach. G. de Gaetano and S. Garattini (eds.) Raven Press: New York, 427-446.

Malignancy and the Hemostatic System,
edited by M. B. Donati et al.
Raven Press, New York © 1981.

Cancer Cell–Endothelial Reactions: The Microinjury Hypothesis and Localized Thrombosis in the Formation of Micrometastases

B. A. Warren

Department of Pathology, University of Western Ontario, London, Ontario, Canada

Currently there are an enormous number of unanswered questions with regard to the biology of the development of metastases from malignant tumors. In this section are presented some work and ideas concerning two stages in the process of the development of metastases viz:

(a) the intravasation of malignant cells in the primary malignant tumor; and,

(b) the factors which build up to arrest and the nature of the arrest of tumor emboli in the circulation and the movement of these cells out of the vascular compartment.

The basic sequence of stages in the development of metastases is shown in Fig. 1. As part of the overall situation affecting the fate of the tumor embolus, those factors operating at the tumor embolus/endothelial surface may play a role of considerable importance. Following the development of the primary tumor there is the movement into the vascular lumen by malignant cells, or intravasation, circulation in the vessels followed by arrest, extravasation and growth in the extravascular site. The process may then once again return to the stage of issuing malignant cells into the bloodstream.

A. THE MOVEMENT OF MALIGNANT TUMOR CELLS INTO THE VASCULAR LUMEN

The first of the significant cancer cell–endothelial reactions is the movement of cancer cells into the vascular lumen. Fig. 2 indicates some of the forces which are operative when a cancer cell penetrates the endothelial lining of a vessel in the primary tumor in order to pass into the lumen of the vessel.

Certain types of vessels, particularly the marginal giant capillaries present at the edge of some tumors, appear to be preferential sites for migration of cells into the vascular lumen (34).

FIG. 1. Factors involved in the formation of metastases via the bloodstream. T = tumor cell; P = blood platelet; E = endothelial cell; BM = basement membrane of endothelium.

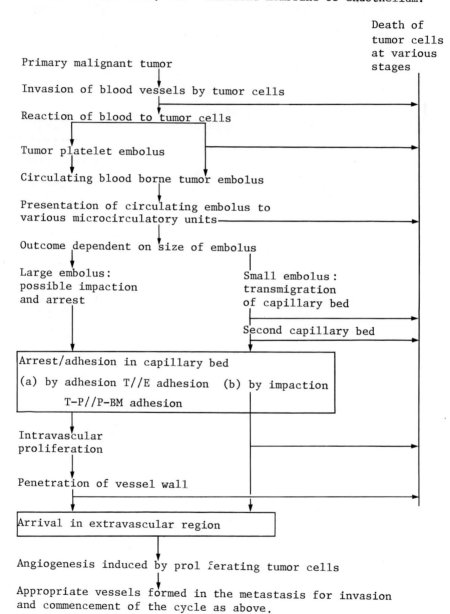

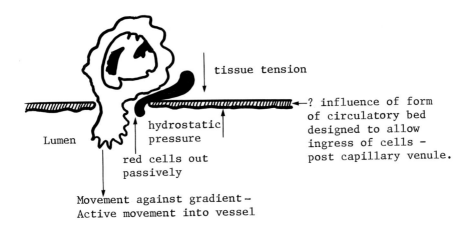

FIG. 2. The forces which are operative when a tumor cell passes into the vascular lumen.

Ultrastructural examination of such vessels have shown single tumor cells in various stages of penetration through the wall (34). The penetration of the wall appears to be composed of a step-wise process in which the opposing barriers are each in turn overcome. The tumor cell first lies close to the basement membrane of the endothelium. The basement membrane then undergoes "lysis" or disintegration in its portion directly between the tumor cell and the endothelium. The basement membrane layer in these vessels is reinforced sporadically with collagen bundles. The structural integrity of these collagen fibers remains and the tumor cell moves through a gap in the basement membrane between sets of reinforcing collagen fibers. The tumor cell moves through in a dumbell fashion, and the nucleus appears less liable to compression and alteration of its form than any other part of the cell. The tumor cell then lies between the endothelial cell layer and its basement membrane. The endothelial cells overlying the tumor cell become thinned out to such an extent that in some cases it is difficult to determine whether the next stage involves dis-integration of the thin layer or separation at an endothelial cell junction. The tumor cell plasmalemmal membrane next moves through the gap produced in the endothelial cell layer and is seen in redundant folds within the vascular lumen. Cytoplasmic contents flow into the redundant folds of the plasmalemmal membrane and the cytoplasm fills up the redundant plasmalemmal membrane in the lumen. Part of the nucleus may be among the few remaining structures left in the endothelial cell gap which provides the attachment of the now mostly luminal tumor

cell to the vessel wall. Soon this is also withdrawn and the
tumor cell floats freely in the lumen of the vessel.

Small platelet aggregates attached to damaged regions of
the vessel wall are sometimes found in these vessels and may
represent platelet adhesion to former regions of entry of tumor
cells. This sequence of changes in transplantable hamster
melanoma is indicative of active movement of tumor cells into
the lumen (34). In this process of intravasation the tumor
cells move into the lumen singly and not together in groups.

This type of route into the circulation has been
observed by means of both transmission and scanning electron
microscopy in subcutaneously implanted Shay acute myelogenous
leukaemic infiltrates (4). In this particular tumor the
malignant cell moved through the bodies of endothelial cells
in venules within the tumor creating a temporary "migration
pore" (4).

It is recognized that what has been shown as a route of
entrance of malignant cells into the bloodstream in a particular
class of tumor vessel may not have general applicability. However, the size of the tumor cell embolus appears linked to its
mode of origin. Large masses may break off a column of renal
carcinoma cells growing along a renal vein into the inferior
vena cava; whereas intravasation of tumor cells into an
internal tumor microcirculatory bed which possesses deficiencies
is likely to yield micro-emboli of only single cells or a very
small number of cells.

The viability, clonal characteristics and invasiveness
of different component cells in a tumor cell embolus are
likely to vary considerably. Necrosis and death of cells are
part of the biology of tumors, and, indeed certain tumors
possess a pattern of necrosis which is one of the hallmarks of
the type. Dead cells may occur as part of the embolus and may
themselves aid in attachment by resulting in damage to the
adjacent endothelium, perhaps by causing the contraction of
individual endothelial cells. Examination of the content of
efferent vessels in human renal adenocarcinoma has shown a
mixture of tumor cells, and necrotic debris from degenerating
tumor cells as well as strands of fibrin (30).

Weiss (37) in a series of studies showed that detachment
of viable cancer cells is facilitated by proximity to necrotic
regions in Walker 256 tumors and that extracts from necrotic
material aided their _in vitro_ detachment. This detachment was
partially inhibited by hydrocortisone. He suggested that the
extracts acted by labilizing the W-256 cell lysosomes, and
emphasizes the importance of reference to specific regions of
the same tumor when reference is made to its metastatic and
other properties. The extract of necrotic material was prepared
by curetting out the necrotic centres of W-256 tumors and
rinsing the tumors with 145 mM NaCl at 4°C, then pooling the
material and homogenizing it.

Liotta et al (15) showed that with the T241 fibrosarcoma metastases were first observed on Day 10 and increased at a rate similar to that of the concentration of tumor cell clumps of 4 or more cells in the effluent from the tumor. In further work (16) this group found that injection of tumor cells in clumps of 6 or 7 cells produced a significantly greater number of metastatic foci than did a similar number of single tumor cells. It was found on injection of radioactively labelled cells about 5% of the tumor cells injected were retained in the lung in micrometastases and their average death rate could be monitored by loss of radioactivity (17).

The size of emboli of malignant cells is dependent not only upon the number of component cells but also upon the size of the individual cells and malignant cells are usually much larger than polymorphonuclear leucocytes. Saccomanno (23) has studied the size of cells exfoliated from primary and secondary malignant neoplasms of the lung. He used the techniques of exfoliative cytology in which, because the preparations are smears and the whole cell is seen in a single preparation, it is much easier to make firm measurements concerning the sizes of cells. This is in contrast to paraffin embedded material in which only "profiles" of cells are seen because of the section-thickness of about 8 microns. Cells from primary bronchogenic malignancies range in size from a low of 8-20 microns for small cell undifferentiated carcinoma to cells of 200 microns in the giant cell undifferentiated carcinomas of the lung. Cells of the keratinizing epidermoid carcinoma are about 100 microns in diameter.

The diameters of adenocarcinoma cells from secondary deposits in the lung were large when compared with normal blood cells. Examples are cells from metastases from adenocarcinoma of breast (intraduct type) 30 to 50 microns in diameter, adenocarcinoma of pancreas 50 to 80 microns in diameter and adenocarcinoma of large bowel 12 to 35 microns in diameter.

Except for the lower range of values given for the small cell carcinoma of the lung, these measurements are all much larger, sometimes by a considerable factor than the 10 to 12 microns that a normal human neutrophil measures in diameter (18).

A group of adenocarcinoma cells from a bronchogenic tumor is depicted in Fig. 3. Even the individual malignant cells in the group, despite some variation in size, are much larger than the polymorphs.

Platelets react to the plasmalemmal surfaces of certain tumor cells as they would react to a foreign surface and undergo shape change with the production of pseudopodia similar to that shown in Fig. 4.

Platelet aggregation can be induced by certain tumor lines and this is usually species specific (7) and may occur only with particular tumors, i.e. this property is not necessarily linked to specific histologic types.

Platelets so activated may act as the cohesive binding single tumor cells together and so creating a platelet-tumor body of considerable size (27).

FIG. 3. Group of adenocarcinoma cells from a malignant tumor of the lung. The large cells are adenocarcinoma cells. The smaller cells are polymorphs and macrophages (X 500).

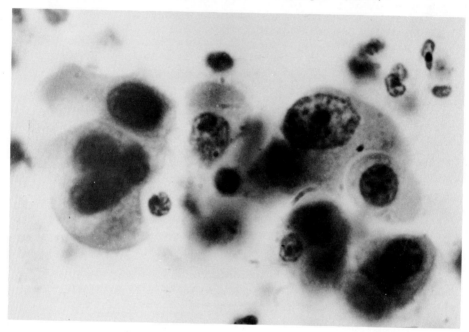

FIG. 4. Activated platelets adhering to uncoated glass.
Each platelet has put out a number of pseudopodia. The white
bars are each one micron in length.

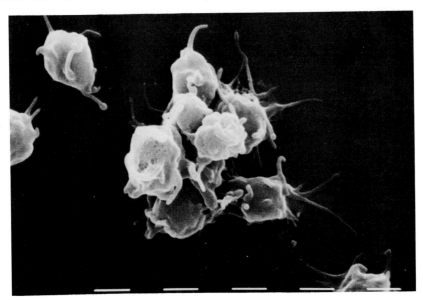

        The shedding characteristics of tumors are likely to be
interwoven with the maturation of their vascular supply and
their vascular morphology, which has been reviewed elsewhere
(31). There are a number of possible variations in geometric
patterns within the framework of connections between the
circulatory systems of host and tumor for example:

1. Arteriole – capillary sprouts – capillary bed – venule
      of host   in tumor   of host

2. Arteriole – capillary bed – capillary bed – venule
                of host   of tumor   of host

3. Arteriole – capillary bed – capillary bed – "veins" – venules
                of host   of tumor   of tumor   of host

4. Arteriole – capillary bed – venules – capillary bed – venules
                       of host   of tumor   of host
        Important parts of the biology of the metastatic process
for each malignant tumor are the shedding characteristics and
the wastage of tumor cells in the circulation (Fig. 5).

FIG. 5.   Some quantitative estimates of the shedding characteristics of tumors and the survival of malignant cells in the
circulation.

Primary tumor

10^6 cells per gram of adenocarcinoma shed into
blood in rat per day (2).

Mechanical damage and death removes majority of
cells (5).   (B16 Melanoma cells)

	of 200,000	^{125}IUdR labelled B16 cells injected
only	136,000	" viable at 1 min.
	108,000	" at 1 hr.
	5,500	" at 12 hr.
	355	" at 14 days.

A.   FACTORS INVOLVED IN THE ARREST OF TUMOR CELLS IN THE
     CIRCULATION

     Wastage of circulating tumor cells is of a very high
order, (Fig. 6), before even a single metastasis is produced.
Tumor embolism is not tumor metastasis and this has been shown
repeatedly in the cancer research literature and in man in
a series of studies in the 1960s notably those of Ritchie and
Webster (1961) (21) and Goldblatt and Nadel (1963 and 1965)
(10,11). Ritchie and Webster found that in the great
majority of patients with breast carcinoma, malignant cells
were present in the blood at some time. It was concluded that
the presence of tumor cells in the blood did not provide a
clear cut marker for either prognostic or therapeutic guidance
and the practice of examination of blood for malignant cells
in man has largely been discontinued.

FIG. 6.   The wastage of circulating tumor cells.

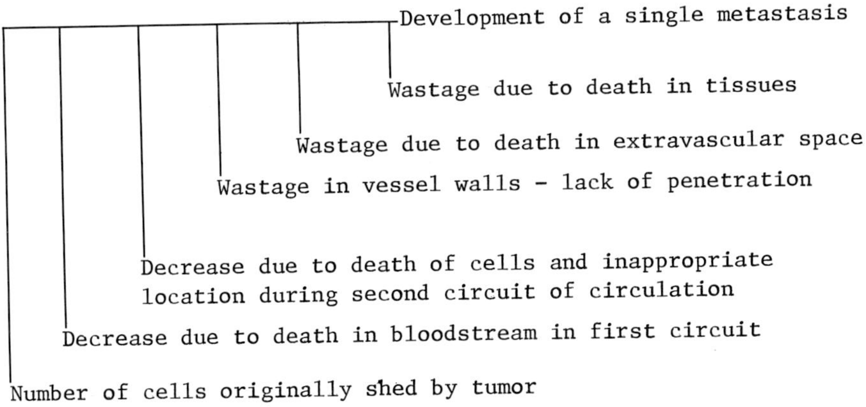

```
                                    ┌─Development of a single metastasis
 ┌───────┬───────┬───────┬──────────┤
 │       │       │       │          └Wastage due to death in tissues
 │       │       │       └─Wastage due to death in extravascular space
 │       │       └─Wastage in vessel walls - lack of penetration
 │       │
 │       └─Decrease due to death of cells and inappropriate
 │         location during second circuit of circulation
 └─Decrease due to death in bloodstream in first circuit
Number of cells originally shed by tumor
```

Kinjo (14) described three types of tumor cell emboli in the arterioles and capillaries of the lungs following injection of three types of ascites hepatoma cells. The first type consisted of marked aggregation of platelets associated with detachment of endothelial cells (tumor cells with high thromboplastic activity), the second type had only loosely aggregated platelets and the third type was free of platelets and fibrin. Possible variations in the composition of the blood borne tumor embolus are listed in Fig. 7.

The interaction between endothelium and cancer cells is a focal point of the metastasis problem (1,35). Studies of collisions between circulating cells and endothelium have been made (12) and the different aspects of the surface components of cells (20) and the interactions between normal and malignant cells reviewed (35). The complexity of the situation is increased in the consideration of adhesion of the blood borne tumor embolus to the vessel wall because of the interposition of the reaction of the blood both to the tumor embolus itself and to any alteration from normal that the endothelial lining of the wall may show. The adhesion of platelets and the effects of altered surfaces in hemostasis and thrombosis without the interposition of tumor embolism is not simple (24).

FIG. 7.   Possible variations in the components of the blood borne tumor embolus.

    (a)   The tumor cells
           ? multiplying
           ? dying
           ? associated products
           ? associated debris

    (b)   Reaction of blood to foreign surfaces of substances under (a)

          1.   Nature of surface and adsorbed plasma protein

          2.   Platelet adhesion to certain tumor cells

In any consideration of the development of metastases from circulating tumor emboli three separate elements must be brought into focus: (1) the tumor cells themselves; (2) the reaction of the blood to the tumor cell surfaces and (3) the endothelial surface of the blood vessels. Much important information concerning the function and biochemical attributes of endothelial cells has been published in recent years. The vascular endothelial cell is a major source of plasminogen activator although the control mechanisms of activator release are still under investigation (3). Plasminogen activator converts the inactive precursor plasminogen to the active protease, plasmin which lyses fibrin.

Gimbrone has reviewed the harvesting of endothelium from large vessels (8) and the metabolism within endothelial cells of such vasoactive agents as prostaglandins and angiotensin (9). Cultured endothelial cells occur as simple monolayers and require higher (by severalfold) serum concentrations of mitogenic factors than vascular smooth muscle cells for the same effect. Cell replication and migration after interruption of the mono-layer by mechanical injury have been observed with reconstitution of the confluence of the monolayer. A prostaglandin synthetase which is sensitive to indomethacin is found in cultured endothelial cells. There is an interplay between substances within platelets and those within the endothelium. The stimulation of platelets to aggregate forms prostaglandin endoperoxide. In the absence of endothelium, this substance can remain within the platelet and be converted to thromboxane A_2. This decreases the cyclic AMP levels and promotes platelet aggregation and vasoconstriction. In the presence of endoth-elium prostaglandin endoperoxide escapes from the platelets and

is utilized by prostacyclin synthetase in the vessel wall.
Prostacyclin (prostaglandin I_2) is released and taken up by
the platelets where the platelet cyclic AMP is raised and hence
platelet aggregation is inhibited. Prostacyclin acts as a
vasodilator (19).

A renin-like enzyme and angiotensin I converting enzyme
(Kininase II) which act as part of the renin-angiotensin system
have been found in cultured endothelial cells. Endothelial
cells can generate from a synthetic renin precursor angiotensin
I which they can then convert to its active pressor form,
angiotensin II. Other associated actions are the release of
prostaglandin E following stimulation by angiotensin and the
degradation of bradykinin (26).

Allied to the type of reaction to the endothelial
surface is the nature of the organization of the vessels in the
smallest of the microcirculatory units. The anatomy of the
microcirculatory modules of organs may play a vital role from
the point of view of the opportunity presented to the circulating
tumor embolus for plugging for prolonged periods the entrance
vessel or vessels to these units. Determining factors in the
ability of tumor emboli to plug these vessels would include
the presence or absence of encrusted platelets and fibrin, the
deformability and size of the tumor cells themselves and the
number of cells in the embolus.

The Microinjury Hypothesis of Organ Retention of Malignant Cells

This hypothesis suggests that showers of tumor emboli
discharged into a capillary system repeatedly plug the entrance
to capillary beds. Anoxic degeneration of the endothelium of
portions of the capillary network then ensues and such areas
provide preferential adhesion sites for circulating tumor
emboli (13). The variations in structure in different organs
of the smallest units of the microcirculation (the microcirculatory modules) are vital determinants in the development of
metastases within the framework of this hypothesis of the
formation of metastases.

There are diverse local injuries to tissues which result
in an increase in the number of metastases from circulating
tumor cells at the site of injury (for review see 22, 32) and
our earlier work is highly supportive of the concept that an
injured vessel wall allows a more ready attachment at that site
for circulating tumor cells (28,29,32,33). It is apparent that
the progress through the vessel wall and the arrest of tumor
cells within the lumen depends upon the interaction of tumor
cells and the endothelial lining with its adjacent basement
membrane together with the intervention of constituents of
the blood stream.

How these multiple forms of injury are translated into
increased metastatic deposits is not at all clear although the

suggestion that endothelial injury is involved as a common factor has been made. Direct local injury in vitro to endothelial cells results in the provision of bare basement membrane to which malignant cells will adhere (Fig. 8) (32).

Indirect local injury in vivo especially where the endothelium shows intracellular fenestrations aids in attachment of tumor cells (Fig. 9a and b).

FIG. 8. Electron micrograph of a HeLa cell (H) adhering directly to the subendothelial layer (S) of human vein wall. This is from an in vitro preparation in which the endothelial surface of human vein wall (removed at saphenous vein stripping) was damaged and a suspension of HeLa cells added to it (32) (X 10,000).

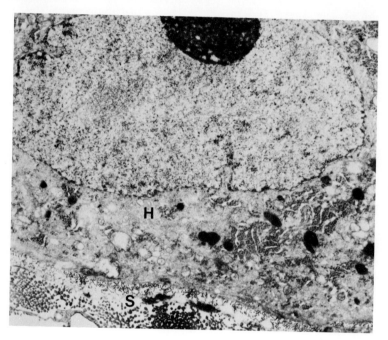

FIG. 9. Low (Fig. 9a) and high (Fig. 9b) power views of a
Walker 256 tumor cell adherent to the endothelial lining of
a glomerular tuft in a rat kidney. 0.1 ml of air was injected
into the artery of the left kidney of an anaesthetized rat and
3 min. later 0.1 ml of a suspension of Walker 256 tumor cells
was injected.

(a) This electron micrograph shows a Walker 256 tumor
cell (W) occluding the lumen of a glomerular tuft. Processes
of podocytes (P) are present on the outer aspect of the basement
membrane of the capillary. Microvilli of the tumor cell are
attached through the fenestrae of the glomerular endothelial
cell to the basement membrane. The region indicated by an
arrow is shown at higher power in Fig. 9b   (X 7,200).

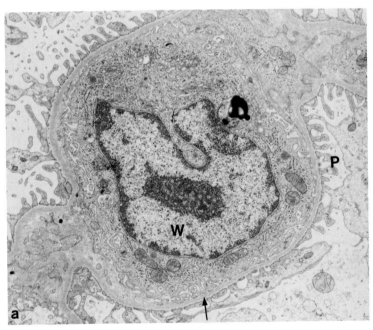

FIG. 9b. Microvilli of the Walker 256 tumor cell (M1,M2,M3) are close or adherent to the basement membrane (BM) of the glomerular capillary, and interdigitate with portions of the endothelial cytoplasm   (X 33,100).

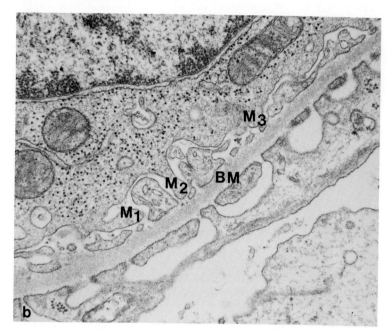

The microinjury hypothesis suggests a way in which tumor cell showers passing through a microcirculatory bed may so injure the capillary units that they are more receptive to the next tumor shower.

In Fig. 10 one circulatory bed is shown at different times in diagrammatic form.

FIG. 10. Diagrams illustrating the microinjury hypothesis of organ retention of tumor cells.

(a) Tumor cell emboli (TE1) in the arterial system pass into the main arteriole (MA) leading to a capillary bed. Tumor cell emboli (TE2, TE3, TE4) become impacted in the arteriolar branches at the precapillary sphincter regions leading into the capillary bed. This eventually results in anoxic damage to a distal region of the capillary bed (D). The venule (V) drains this capillary bed.

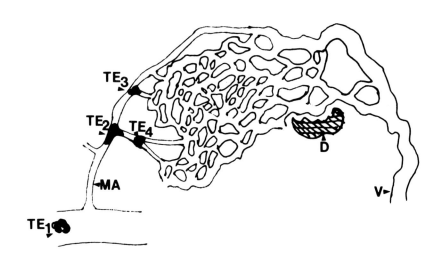

a

FIG. 10b. Adhesion of tumor cells to the damaged area occurs
either when the emboli (TE2, TE3 and TE4) flow through the
capillary bed or when the capillary bed is open, from subsequent
emboli. Progression through the wall is aided by the fact that
this region has suffered from anoxic damage. There results a
micrometastasis (M) near the site of injury.

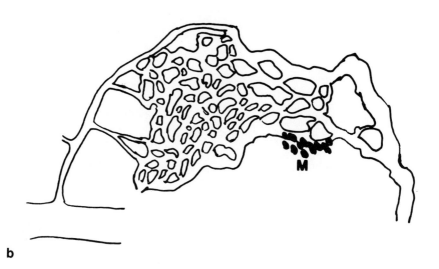

b

Tumor cells may pass without hindrance through the
capillary bed if they are small and single or they may obstruct
the capillary bed for a prolonged time if they are large. It is
suggested that the site of obstruction would occur at the precapillary sphincter and that the site of microinjury due to
hypoxia following stasis would be at the venular end of the
capillary bed.

Occasionally in vivo in thin preparations one can see
leucocytes blocking the entrances to capillary beds. In the case
of tumor emboli this plugging may result in significant damage
to some sites of the capillary bed and this is the microinjury
involved.

On unplugging or uncorking the system the blood flows
again through the area and brings to the injured area fresh
tumor emboli. These new emboli adhere to the site of the

microinjury and because of the injury the damaged wall allows transit from the lumen to the extravascular position more readily than it otherwise would have done.

The shedding characteristics of the malignant tumor are important from the viewpoint both of the number of tumor cells shed and whether or not they are in clumps and the number of cells in each clump.

The possible fates of the tumor cell emboli are transit, disintegration and finally blockage with penetration or impaction with attrition of the endothelium.

The microinjury hypothesis of the induction of receptive areas for the transmural passage of tumor cells is consistent with present information regarding the release into the circulation of showers of tumor cells from primary or secondary deposits of malignant tumors.

In the study by Kawaguchi and Nakamura (13) they found that:

1. "Island–forming" strains of tumors (AH–130, AH–272 and AH–7974) resulted in low cerebral passage rate and metastatic foci.

2. Single cell strains (Yoshida sarcoma, AH–7974F, AH–66F and AH–13) showed high rates of transcerebral passage and no metastases.

They concluded that the incidence of metastases corresponds directly to the frequency of arrested tumor cells in some models (13). The microinjury hypothesis was based on their own work and the following pertinent observations by Sato and others (25) and Fujikura (6):
(a) Transient circulating tumor cells in arterioles and metarterioles may result in functional disturbance of the microcirculation (25), and
(b) Tissue injury can occur from tumor embolism (6).

The factors involved in the arrest of tumor cells in the microcirculation are summarized in Fig. 11.

FIG. 11.   Summary of the factors involved in the arrest of
           tumor cells.

Primary tumor

? Constant shedding
of tumor emboli –
probably dependent upon
type and stage of tumor

Repeated showers of emboli
in transit through capillary
beds with arrest due to:

1. Factors dependent on embolus

    (a) size ± platelets

    (b) deformability

    (c) effect on endothelium

2. Factors determined by pattern
    of circulation and vessel wall
    morphology

    (a) next capillary bed

    (b) by-pass routes

    (c) damage to vessel wall

     Further information as to the composition of the tumor
embolus, the nature of the process of arrest of tumor emboli,
the migration of tumor cells through the vessel wall and the
factors concerned with their survival or death in the
immediately extravascular site would provide important leads
to the processes vulnerable to therapeutic attack in the prevention of the spread of this disease via the bloodstream. If
the microinjury hypothesis is correct then measures which
support endothelial and vessel wall integrity may aid both in
reducing the number of cells entering the blood within the
primary tumor and help to prevent attachment and metastasis.

SUMMARY

Although tumor cells have been demonstrated in blood, it has not been possible to correlate prognosis with the occurrence or absence of tumor cells in the blood. Nevertheless, metastasis via the bloodstream is an important mode of dissemination of tumors and in some way circulating tumor emboli do implant and eventually form metastases. The principal distinguishing features of those emboli which will progress to form metastasis are unknown although it is suggested by some animal work that the larger the tumor embolus involved, the more likely it is to eventually form a metastatic deposit. Many tumor cells induce platelet aggregation when mixed with blood but this relationship is far from simple in that the reaction of tumor cells in this respect is almost specific for the individual tumor and only general tendencies can be surmized from the histology of the tumor. Although "tumor embolism is not tumor metastasis", arrest of the embolus is closely linked to metastasis formation, and injury to tissues results in preferential location of metastases in those injured tissues from circulating cells. Much of the current work is consistent with the Microinjury Hypothesis and the concept that there is localized thrombosis at the site of injury. This hypothesis suggests that blockage for varying periods of the microcirculatory unit by repeated showers of embolic tumor cells so injures regions of the capillary network within the unit that a site for preferential attachment is presented to the circulating tumor cells.

The support of the National Cancer Institute of Canada is gratefully acknowledged.

REFERENCES

1. Born, G.V.R. (1978): In *Platelets: A Multidisciplinary Approach*, edited by G. de Gaetano and S. Garattini, p. 419, Raven Press, New York.
2. Butler, T.P. and Gullino, P.M. (1975): *Cancer Res.*, **35**, 512.
3. Cash, J.D. (1978): In *Progress in Chemical Fibrinolysis and Thrombolysis*, vol. 3, edited by J.F. Davidson et al., p. 65, Raven Press, New York.
4. De Bruyn, P.P.H. and Cho, Y. (1979): *J. Nat. Cancer Inst.*, **62**, 1221
5. Fidler, I.J. (1976): In *Fundamental Aspects of Metastasis*, edited by L. Weiss, p. 275, North Holland, Amsterdam.
6. Fujikura, T., Isomura, S., Kawaai, S. (1972): *Nippon Byôri Gakkai Kaishi*, **61**, 141, cited by Kawaguchi and Nakamura,1977 (13).
7. Gasic, G.J., Boettiger, D., Catalfamo, J.L., Gasic, T.B. and Stewart, G.J. (1978): In *Platelets: A Multidisciplinary Approach*, edited by G. de Gaetano and S. Garattini,

   p. 447, Raven Press, New York.
8. Gimbrone, M.A. Jr. (1976): In Progress in Haemostasis and
   Thrombosis, vol. 3, edited by T.H. Spaet, p. 1, Grune
   and Stratton, New York.
9. Gimbrone, M.A. Jr. (1977): In International Cell Biology
   1976–1977, edited by B.D. Brinkley and K.R. Porter,
   p. 649, Rockefeller University Press, New York.
10. Goldblatt, S.A. and Nadel, E.M. (1963): In Cancer Progress,
    edited by R.W. Raven, p. 119, Butterworths, London.
11. Goldblatt, S.A. and Nadel, E.M. (1965): Acta Cytol. 9, 6.
12. Goldsmith, H.L. (1976): In Fundamental Aspects of
    Metastasis, edited by L. Weiss, p. 99, North Holland,
    Amsterdam.
13. Kawaguchi, T. and Nakamura, K. (1977): Gann 68, 65.
14. Kinjo, M. (1978): Br. J. Cancer, 38, 293.
15. Liotta, L.A., Kleinerman, J. and Saidel, G.M. (1974):
    Cancer Res. 34, 997.
16. Liotta, L.A., Kleinerman, J. and Saidel, G.M. (1976):
    Cancer Res. 36, 889.
17. Liotta, L.A., Vembu, D., Saini, R.K. and Boone, C. (1978):
    Cancer Res. 38, 1231.
18. Matthews, J.L. and Martin, J.H. (1971): In Atlas of Human
    Histology and Ultrastructure, Lea and Febiger,
    Philadelphia, p. 82.
19. Moncada, S. and Vane, J.R. (1978): In British Medical
    Bulletin: Thrombosis, vol. 34, edited by D. Thomas,
    p. 129.
20. Revel, J.P. and Ito, S. (1967): In The Specificity of Cell
    Surfaces, edited by B.D. Davis and L. Warren, p. 211,
    Prentice–Hall, New Jersey.
21. Ritchie, A.C. and Webster, D.R. (1961): In Canadian Cancer
    Conference, edited by R.W. Begg et al., p. 225, Academic
    Press, New York.
22. Rudenstam, C.M. (1968): Experimental Studies on Trauma and
    Metastasis Formation, supplement 391, Acta Chir. Scandinav.,
    Stockholm, Sweden.
23. Saccomanno, G., (1978): Diagnostic Pulmonary Cytology,
    American Society of Clinical Pathologists.
24. Salzman, E. (1972): In The Chemistry of Biosurfaces, Vol. 2,
    edited by M.L. Hair, p. 489, Marcel Dekker, New York.
25. Sato, H., Suzuki, M., Kurokawa, Y. (1967): Kōsankinbyo
    Kenkyu Zasshi 19, 2, cited by Kawaguchi and Nakamura,
    1977 (13).
26. Smith, U. and Ryan, J.W. (1972): Adv. exp. Med. Biol. 21,
    267.
27. Warren, B.A. (1970): Br. J. exp. Pathol. 51, 570.
28. Warren, B.A. (1973): J. Med. 4, 150.
29. Warren, B.A. (1976) Z. Krebsforsch. 87, 1.

30. Warren, B.A. (1978): In Platelets: A Multidisciplinary Approach, edited by G. de Gaetano and S. Garattini, p. 427, Raven Press, New York.
31. Warren, B.A. (1979): In Tumor Blood Circulation: Angiogenesis, Vascular Morphology and Blood Flow of Experimental and Human Tumors, chapter 1, edited by H.I. Peterson, CRC Press, Florida, (In Press).
32. Warren, B.A. and Güldner, F.H. (1969): Angiologica 6, 32.
33. Warren, B.A. and Vales, O. (1972): Br. J. exp. Pathol. 53, 301.
34. Warren, B.A., Shubik, P. and Feldman, R. (1978): Cancer Let. 4, 245.
35. Weiss, L. (1972): In The Chemistry of Biosurfaces, Vol. 2, edited by M.L. Hair, p. 377, Marcel Dekker, New York.
36. Weiss, L. (1977): Seminars in Oncology 4, 5.
37. Weiss, L. (1978): Int. J. Cancer 22, 196.

Malignancy and the Hemostatic System,
edited by M. B. Donati et al.
Raven Press, New York © 1981.

In Vitro Mechanism of Platelet Aggregation by Purified Plasma Membrane Vesicles Shed by Mouse 15091A Tumor Cells

Gabriel J. Gasic, James L. Catalfamo, Tatiana B. Gasic
and Nebojsa Avdalovic*

*Department of Pathology, University of Pennsylvania School of Medicine, and the
Wistar Institute,* Philadelphia, Pennsylvania 19104*

Previous work has demonstrated that primary rat embryo
cells transformed in vitro by Rous Sarcoma virus induced
the aggregation of rat platelets in vitro (3). The aggregating activity was shown to be specific for the transformed
cells and was absent in the normal parent cells. The
aggregation reaction was accompanied by the release of
serotonin from the platelets. Further analysis and purification of this activity from the transformed cells demonstrated that the activity was shed from cells growing in
culture and was associated with membrane vesicles of hetero-
geneous sizes. Normal cells also produce vesicles in culture, however, the level of vesicle production was less
than that from transformed cells and the platelet aggregation and serotonin releasing activities were greatly
reduced or absent in these vesicles.

The capacity of shedded vesicles to aggregate platelets
was also observed in established mouse tumor cell lines,
such as MCA6, a methylcholanthrene-induced sarcoma (4), and
15091A, which is a mouse spontaneous mammary adenocarcinoma
(4), both kept as ascites tumors. Since vesicles shed by
these tumor cells can easily be collected, this material was
used to investigate the mechanism of platelet aggregation
induced by tumor vesicles. Furthermore, electron microscopic
studies (14), external iodination of cells, and analysis of
enzyme markers of the cell membrane (to be published), have
established that vesicles shed by 15091A cells derive from the
plasma membrane.

Vesicles were collected from free viable 15091A cells, washed
and resuspended in Dulbecco's modified Eagle medium. After
incubation at 37°C for one hour in a rotary shaker at 80 rpm,
cells were pelleted by centrifugation and the plasma membrane
vesicles separated from cytoplasmic particles by sucrose
density gradient centrifugation, as previously described (3).
The activity of the separated fractions were tested for

platelet aggregation (PA) in an aggregometer by adding different amounts of the fraction suspended in 50 μl of PBS to 450 μl heparinized rat platelet rich plasma (PRP).

The fraction containing purified vesicles was the most active, causing irreversible aggregation with as little as one microgram of vesicular protein. The aggregation was preceded by a lag of 1 or more minutes depending on the protein concentration in the fraction. The higher the concentration, the shorter the lag period.

PA by this material could be due to direct activation of platelets by physical adhesion of vesicles (binding), to activation of a plasma factor, or to a more complex mechanism involving the three components of the in vitro system.

To investigate whether vesicle binding is a prerequisite for PA, plasma membrane vesicles from mouse 15091A tumor cells were labelled with ^{125}I (6), added to heparinized rat PRP, and samples of the mixture taken at different stages of PA, as indicated by arrows in Figure 1. The measurements of radioactivity after centrifugation indicate that most of the radioactivity present in the pellet was bound to platelets (Table 1). This binding precedes PA (Table 1, first line), suggesting that PA may involve two sequential stages: a first stage of vesicle binding and a second stage of PA; binding also occurs when aggregation was blocked by prostacyclin (Table 1, fourth line). Trappings of ^{125}I-labelled vesicles by platelet aggregates had little additive effect on the radioactivity associated with the pellet of platelets, as shown by the second and third lines of Table 1.

To determine the role of plasma in vesicle binding, platelets were free from plasma by gel filtration, and their reactivity to tumor vesicles studied. Under these conditions, neither binding nor PA occurred (Table 2, third line). However, if a small aliquot of heparinized rat plasma is added back to the system, binding took place and aggregation proceeded in the usual fashion (Table 2, fourth line), indicating that plasma cofactors were instrumental in both events.

Since heating of rat plasma at 56°C for 30 minutes abolished the capacity of rat plasma to support binding (Table 3, second line), our attention was directed toward complement.

Using complement deficient plasmas or sera from different species, it was found that binding:

(1) Does not occur if guinea pig component 4 is absent from the complement system (Table 4, first and second lines). The

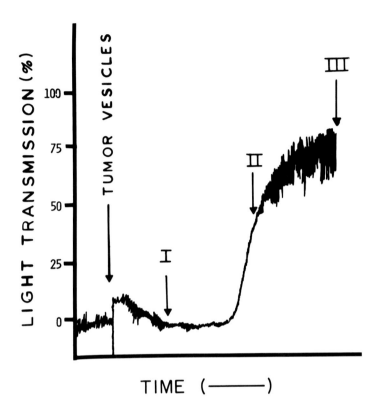

FIG. 1. PA by radiolabelled vesicles shed by mouse 15091A tumor cells. Addition of tumor vesicles (first arrow) is followed by a lag period and then by irreversible PA. Arrows with Roman numbers indicate times at which samples were taken for radio-labelled vesicle binding studies.

binding is partially restored, however, if purified guinea pig complement component 4, or guinea pig plasma heated at 56°C for 30 minutes, is added to C4-deficient guinea pig serum (Table 4, fourth and fifth lines). Heating of plasma inactivates termolabile components, except components 3 and 4. The latter two, in the absence of other components of the complement system, did not support binding (Table 4, third line).

(2) Is not inhibited by the absence of complement component 5 in mouse plasma as obtained from genetically C5-deficient B10D2 oSN mice (11).

TABLE 1.   Radioactivity specifically bound to platelets at various stages of PA induced by ^{125}I-labelled tumor vesicles[a]

Samples taken in stage	PGI$_2$	PA (%)	Percentage of radio-activity bound to platelets[b] Mean ± S.E.M.	
I	–	0	59 ± 3	(3)
II	–	40	65[c]	(2)
III	–	80	60 ± 4[c]	(3)
IV	+	0	54	(2)

[a]50 µl of radiolabelled vesicles containing 20 µg of proteins were added to 450 µl of heparinized rat PRP and samples from independent assays taken at various stages of PA, or when PA was blocked by PCI$_2$, then centrifuged at 8,000 x g for 15 sec., and radioactivity monitored in the pellet and supernate.

[b]After deducting from the total pelleted radioactivity 25% radioactivity due to sedimentation of radiolabelled vesicles in platelet free plasma.

[c]Radioactivity due to trapping of radiolabelled vesicles by platelet aggregates was not deducted.

[d]Final concentration: 200 nM.

( ) = Number of separate experiments.

TABLE 2.   Capacity of heparinized rat plasma to support vesicle binding and aggregation of rat gel filtered platelets (GFP) by mouse tumor vesicles[a]

GFP	Plasma	Sedimented radio-activity (%)		Specific binding of radiovesicles[b] (%)	Lag (min.)	PA (%)
–	–	26 ± 3	(9)			
–	+	23 ± 0	(5)			
+	–	24 ± 1	(8)	0	–	0
+	+	78 ± 1	(9)	54	3.4 ± 0.2	63 ± 2 (9–14)

[a]For binding studies, 400 µl of GFP or media for their suspension were prewarmed in the aggregometer for 1 min., then 50 µl of plasma or PBS was added followed by the addition of a sub-aggregating dose of 50 µl of the radio-labelled vesicle suspension. After 5 min., the mixture was centrifuged and radioactivity monitored in the pellet and supernate. For aggregation studies, a more concentrated suspension of unlabelled and radiolabelled vesicles were used. Data expressed as Mean and S.E. of the Mean.

[b]After deducting from the total radioactivity in the pellet 24% radioactivity sedimented in the absence of plasma (Third line).

( ) = No. of assays in separate experiments using labelled and unlabelled tumor vesicles, respectively.

TABLE 3. Capacity of heat-treated rat plasma to support binding of radiolabelled vesicles and aggregation of rat GFP[a]

Treatment of plasma	Specific binding of radio- vesicles[b] (%)	Lag (min.)	PA (%)	
Unheated	54 (1)	2.8 ± 0.6	61 ± 4	(8)
Heated, 56°/30 min.	5 (1)	–	0	(1)

[a]Vesicle binding and PA assays are separate, parallel experiments. For binding studies, 400 μl of GFP or media for their suspension were prewarmed in the aggregometer for 1 min., then 50 μl of heated or unheated heparinized plasma were added followed by the addition of sub-aggregating doses of radiolabelled vesicles suspended in PBS. After 5 min., the mixture was centrifuged and radioactivity measured in the pellet and supernate. For aggregation studies, a more concentrated suspension of unlabelled or radiolabelled vesicles was used.
[b]After deducting sedimented radioactivity in the absence of plasma.
[c]Mean and S.E. of the Mean.
( ) = Number of assays in one or more experiments.

TABLE 4. Effect of genetically C4-deficient guinea pig sera and reconstituted mixtures on binding of ^{125}I-labelled vesicles[a]

Guinea pig sera	Percentage of specific ^{125}I-labelled vesicle binding[b]	
1) Normal	39 ± 1[c]	(22)
2) C4-deficient	3 ± 1	(22)
3) Heated, 56°/30 min.	2 ± 0	(10)
4) C4-deficient + C4	34	(2)
5) C4-deficient + heated, 56°/30 min.	23 ± 3	(6)

[a]400 μl of heparinized rat GFP (5 units/ml heparin) were prewarmed in the aggregometer, followed by the addition of 50 μl of normal, C4-deficient, or reconstituted guinea pig sera before the addition of 50 μl of labelled tumor vesicles.
[b]After deducting the percentage of radioactivity due to sedimentation of labelled vesicles in platelet-free media containing aliquots of normal, C4-deficient, or reconstituted guinea pig sera.
[c]Mean and S.E. of the Mean.
( ) = Number of assays in one or more separate experiments.

(3) It is totally suppressed by rat plasma made deficient in complement component 3 by treatment with cobra venom factor (Table 5). Binding was also abolished by EDTA, EGTA, or Mg-EGTA at the final concentration of 9 mM.

TABLE 5. Binding of ^{125}I-labelled mouse tumor vesicles and PA-induced by unlabelled vesicles in C3-deficient rat PRP[a]

Rat PRP	Prothrombin clotting time (sec.)	Specific ^{125}I-vesicle binding (%)	Lag (min.)	PA (%)
Normal	27	62	0.6	86
C3-depleted[c]	27	5	-	0

[a]Data on binding and aggregation from two parallel, separate experiments.
[b]In 1/10 diluted plasma.
[c]Depleted by cobra venom factor (5 units/ml).

The above data strongly suggest the participation of complement in vesicle binding. Since component 4 is required but not component 5, and both calcium and magnesium are needed (2), binding appears as mediated by the activation of the classical pathway (10), but involving only the first four complement components, as in the case of immunoadherence (1,5,12).

Although complement is a prerequisite for vesicle binding, complement alone does not support platelet aggregation. This was demonstrated by adding to gel filtered rat platelets heparinized plasma from coumadin-treated rats. Prothrombin times of these plasmas were at least three times longer than those of normal plasmas. Using plasma from coumadin-treated animals, binding occurs, but not platelet aggregation (Table 6), suggesting that in addition to complement, vitamin K-dependent plasma proteins are needed for platelet aggregation to occur.

These two events, vesicle binding and platelet aggregation, appear to be sequentially linked, as shown by experiments in which binding is abolished by addition of C3-deficient rat plasma to rat gel filtered platelets. In this case, neither binding nor platelet aggregation occurred (Table 5).

Since plasma from coumadin-treated rats does not allow PA, one of the vitamin K-dependent plasma proteins (13) appears to be

TABLE 6. Cofactor activity of plasma from normal and coumadin-treated rats using rat GFP and mouse tumor vesicles[a]

Plasma	Prothrombin clotting time[b] (sec.)	Specific binding of ^{125}I-vesicles (%)	Lag (min.)	PA (5)
Normal	14.3 ±0.2 (3)[c]	57	4.2	55 (2)
Coumadin	42.8 ±0.1 (3)	57	–	0 (2)

[a]Plasma from normal and coumadin-treated rats were collected using heparin as anticoagulant (10 units per ml of whole blood). To 400 μl of rat GFP, prewarmed to 37°C, 50 μl of either normal or coumadinized plasma was added, followed by the addition of 50 μl of vesicles.
[b]For the prothrombin clotting time assays, blood from the same animals was collected and anticoagulated with 3.8% sodium citrate (1 part citrate to 9 parts blood).
[c]Mean and S.E. of the Mean.
( ) = Number of separate experiments.

involved in this phenomenon. With the exception of thrombin, all other vitamin K-dependent plasma proteins, including Protein C (7), most probably do not participate in PA by tumor vesicles. Thus, the most likely plasma protein is thrombin, which at very low doses causes PA but not clotting. To test this possibility, hirudin, a specific and irreversible inhibitor of thrombin (9) was added to heparinized PRP (10 units of heparin per ml) prior to the addition of tumor vesicles. In dose response experiments, it was found that the increasing doses of hirudin prolonged the lag period until a level of hirudin is reached (80 units per ml) that completely abolished PA (Table 7). Similar results were also obtained with heparin, a less specific inhibitor of thrombin (Table 7). We have also studied the effect of diisopropyl fluorophosphate (DFP), an irreversible modifier of serine residues in thrombin and other serine proteases of the clotting system (8), on PA by mouse tumor vesicles. Addition of this inhibitor to heparinized PRP to a final concentration of 5.5 to 16.7 mM, prior to addition of vesicles, almost completely abolished PA. Since this treatment neither modified the capacity of platelets in PRP to respond to collagen or ADP nor the ability of tumor vesicles to induce PA, the abolishing effect of DFP on PA appears to be mediated through serine proteases of the plasma system.

TABLE 7. Effect of thrombin inhibitors on PA by mouse tumor
vesicles using heparinized rat PRP[a]

Inhibitor	Final concentration (units per ml)	Lag (min.)	PA (%)
Heparin[c]	8	1.7 ± 0.1	91 ± 1[b] (4)
	20	2.7 ± 0.1	88 ± 3 (3)
	40	–	0
Hirudin	0	2.7 ± 0.3	87 ± 3 (6)
	20	4.0 ± 0.3	87 ± 3 (6)
	40	5.4 ± 0.1	10 ± 0 (3)
	80	–	0

[a]The assay was performed by adding 50 μl of the inhibitor in
PBS or PBS alone to 400 μl of prewarmed heparinized PRP
(10 units/ml heparin). After 1 min., 50 μl of tumor vesicles
were added and PA recorded by the aggregometer.
[b]Mean and S.E. of the Mean.
[c]Various concentrations of sodium heparin (Sigma) in saline
to a volume of 50 μl were added to 400 μl of heparinized rat PRP
(10 units/ml heparin) to give the final concentration shown by
the Table.
( ) = Number of assays from 1 or more experiments.

These results indicate that PA following vesicle binding might
be due to generation of thrombin. It is tempting to speculate
that vesicles bound to platelets can activate the series of
events leading to generation of thrombin. Once thrombin has been
generated, two different results can be expected. If the amount
of thrombin produced is very low, as when minimal effective doses
of tumor vesicle were added to heparinized PRP, part of the
generated thrombin will be neutralized by the presence of
heparin-antithrombin III complex in the system, and the remaining
free, non-neutralized thrombin will act inducing PA, and the lag
period will depend on the amount of available free thrombin. If
the quantity of thrombin generated is very high, as when
exceptionally high doses of tumor vesicles were used or when
anti-thrombin III was a limiting factor, as when small aliquots
of heparinized plasma were added to GFP, the non-neutralized
portion of thrombin will convert fibrinogen into fibrin following
a variable initial period of PA.

CONCLUSIONS

This study demonstrates that binding of tumor vesicles to platelets precedes platelet aggregation and that two different plasma protein components participate in both events. While binding depends on the activation of the first four components of the complement system, platelet aggregation is probably due to generation of thrombin by the tumor vesicle-platelet complex. Since inhibition of binding prevents platelet-aggregation, these two events might be sequential steps in the mechanism of platelet aggregation induced by tumor plasma membrane vesicles.

ACKNOWLEDGEMENTS

Supported by Grant HL 18827 awarded by U.S. National Heart Lung, and Blood Institute, PHS/DHEW. We thank Drs. Ulm Nillson, Edward P. Kirby, Gwendolyn J. Stewart, Stephan Niewiarowski, Walter Kisiel, and Yale Nemerson for generous gifts of material, suggestions, and criticisms.

REFERENCES

1. Cooper, N.R. (1969): Science, 165: 396-397.
2. Fine, D.P., Marney, S.R., Colley, D.G., Sergent, J.S., and Des Prez, R.M. (1972): J. Immunol., 109: 807-809.
3. Gasic, G.J., Boettiger, D., Catalfamo, J.L., Gasic, T.B., and Stewart, G.J. (1978): Cancer Res., 38: 2950-2955.
4. Gasic, G.J., Gasic, T.B., and Jimenez, S.A. (1977): Lab. Invest., 36: 413-419.
5. Henson, P.M. (1972): In Biological Activities of Complement. Edited by D.G. Ingram, pp. 173-201, S. Karger, New York.
6. Hubbard, A.L., and Cohn, Z.A. (1975): J. Cell Biol., 64: 438-460.
7. Kisiel, W., Canfield, W.M., Ericsson, L.H., and Davie, E.W. (1977): Biochemistry, 16: 5824-5830.
8. Lundblad, R.L., Kingdon, H.S., and Mann, K.G. (1976): Methods in Enzymology, 45: 156-176.
9. Markwardt, F. (1970): Methods in Enzymology, 19: 924-932.
10. Muller-Eberhard, H.J., Hoffman, L.G., Mayer, M.M., Williams, C.A. and Chase, M.W. (1977): In Methods in Immunology and Immunochemistry, Vol. IV. Editors C.A. Williams and M.W. Chase. pp. 127-274. Academic Press, New York.
11. Nilsson, U.R. and Muller-Eberhard, H.J. (1967): J. Exp. Med., 125: 1-16.
12. Nishioka, K. and Linscott, W.D. (1968): J. Exp. Med., 118: 767-793.
13. Stenflo, J. (1978): Advances in Enzymology, 46: 1-31.
14. Stewart, G.J., Gasic, G.J., Gasic, T., Catalfamo, J.L., and Doer, N. (1979): Thrombos. Haemostas, (Stuttgart) 42 (1): 139.

Malignancy and the Hemostatic System,
edited by M. B. Donati et al.
Raven Press, New York © 1981.

The *In Vitro* Activity of Platelet Aggregating Material from SV-40 Transformed Mouse 3T3 Fibroblasts

Simon Karpatkin and Edward Pearlstein

*The Departments of Medicine and Pathology and Irvington House Institute,
New York University Medical School, New York, New York 10016*

SUMMARY

Many tumor cell lines aggregate platelets in vitro, cause thrombocytopenia in vivo, and require platelets for the development of metastases. We have studied the transformed 3T3 mouse fibroblast line, SV3T3. Intact SV3T3 cells aggregate platelets in vitro (heparinized rabbit platelet-rich plasma (PRP)) following a lag period of 1 to 2 min. Untransformed 3T3 cells also aggregate platelets in heparinized PRP but have one-half the activity. SV3T3 cells can be extracted with 1M urea to give a sedimentable (at 100,000 x g) particle which can aggregate rabbit or human platelets at a final concentration of 2.5 μg/ml protein (platelet-aggregating material (PAM)). Extraction of 3T3 cells with 1M urea yields material which barely aggregates platelets at 40 μg/ml. The SV3T3 PAM is inactivated by treatment with neuraminidase, trypsin, phospholipase-A , sonication, non-ionic detergents, and boiling. Phospholipid analysis reveals that the transformed SV3T3 urea extract incorporates 1.8-fold more ^{14}C-oleic acid into phospholipid, 1.9-fold more radioactivity into phosphatidyl serine (PS) and/or phosphatidyl inositol (PI), and 0.6-fold less radioactivity into sphingomyelin than the 3T3 urea extract. PAM induces the platelet release reaction and requires divalent cation, since it releases ^{14}C-serotonin and the aggregation it promotes is inhibited by 5 mM EDTA, 0.5 mM indomethacin, 0.1 mM adenosine, and 0.1 mM N^6, 0$^{2'}$-dibutyrl cyclic AMP. PAM is synergistic with epinephrine-induced aggregation of PRP but not with ADP- or collagen-induced aggregation of PRP. PAM does not aggregate washed platelets in the presence or absence of fibrinogen. However, it can replace the fibrinogen requirement during ADP- or epinephrine-induced platelet aggregation of washed platelets. Addition of platelet-poor plasma (PPP) to the washed platelet system restores PAM's ability to aggregate platelets, thus implicating a plasma factor for PAM activity. We conclude that tumor cells contain a urea-extractable, sedimentable particle which is capable of aggregating platelets via the release reaction in the presence of a plasma factor and divalent cation. Its mechanism

37

of action may be related to its ability to replace fibrinogen as
a supporting medium for washed platelet aggregation with ADP or
epinephrine. PAM is heat-sensitive and requires sialic acid,
phospholipid, and trypsin-sensitive protein constituents for activity. The particle is denatured by non-ionic detergents and
sonication, suggesting that lipid-particle configuration may also
play a role in its activity.

INTRODUCTION

A major problem facing clinicians in the management of malignancies is the ability to prevent or detect distant metastases.
It has previously been demonstrated that tumor cells or media
conditioned by these cells will induce platelet aggregation in
vitro (6,7,10). The significance of this result is apparent in
light of evidence from several laboratories indicating that tumor
cells may also aggregate platelets in vivo (11,15,16,19,37,39,40),
that blood-borne metastases induce thrombocytopenia in the host
(6), that thrombocytopenia impairs the development of metastasis
(9) and that anti-platelet agents alter the metastatic pattern of
tumor spread (8,14). Furthermore, a specific correlation can be
made between in vitro induction of platelet aggregation by various tumor cells and their propensity for lung metastasis (16).
These observations imply a direct role for the platelet in the
pathogenesis of tumor cell metastasis.

In order to define the mechanism of platelet-tumor cell interaction, an in vitro system was developed employing the normal
mouse fibroblast cell line 3T3 as a control and the virally transformed SV3T3 cell line as the tumor cell. A technique has been
established for extracting PAM from the transformed cell. This
PAM has been partially characterized and its mechanism of action
studied.

MATERIALS AND METHODS

Cell Culture

A low passage Balb C/3T3 fibroblast cell line and its SV40
virally transformed derivative (SV3T3) were obtained from stocks
at the Imperial Cancer Research Fund, London, and were maintained
in Dulbecco's Modified Eagle's medium (E4) supplemented with 10%
fetal calf serum, 2 mM glutamine, 100 U/ml penicillin, and 100
μg/ml streptomycin (34). Cells were passaged twice weekly.

Extraction of PAM

Cells were grown to confluency on 10 cm tissue-culture dishes
and washed twice with Veronal buffer (11.75 gm of sodium diethyl
barbiturate, 14.67 gm of sodium chloride, 430 ml of 0.1N HCl,
H_2O to 2 L, final pH 7.4). Three milliliters of 1M urea, dissolved in Veronal buffer, were then added. Dishes were shaken at

30°C for 1 hr in a 5% CO_2 atmosphere, the supernatants were spun at 2000 x g for 5 min to remove any floating cells, and the cell-free supernatant was dialyzed against several changes of Veronal buffer for 2 days at 4°C. (Viability of the adherent cells was greater than 90% as judged by trypan blue exclusion following this treatment.) Following dialysis, the supernatant was concentrated in an Amicon chamber with the use of an XM100 membrane (Amicon Corp., Lexington, Mass.) to 1/100 the volume of 1M urea used in the original extraction (approximately 100 μg/ml protein). In parallel cultures, cells were extracted with E4 or 0.3 mM KCl, and extracts were processed in an identical fashion.

Preparation of PRP and PPP

Rabbits or humans were bled by venipuncture directly into a plastic syringe containing a final concentration of 5 U/ml heparin (preservative-free, Connaught Laboratories, Willowdale, Ont., Canada). PRP was obtained by centrifugation at 150 x g for 5 min at room temperature. PPP was prepared by centrifuging the remaining blood at 2000 x g for 15 min. The PRP was allowed to stand at room temperature for 30 min in tightly capped plastic tubes prior to testing.

Preparation of Washed Human Platelets

Eighteen milliliters of human blood were drawn into 2 ml of 3.8% trisodium citrate. PRP was prepared as described and incubated with 5 mg of apyrase at 37°C for 30 min. The platelets were then sedimented as above and resuspended in Ardlie's buffer (26) containing 0.2 U/ml heparin and 0.5 mg/ml apyrase, except that $MgCl_2$ and $CaCl_2$ were omitted from the buffer and 2 mM EDTA was added. The resuspended platelets were again centrifuged, resuspended in half their original PRP volume of Ardlie's buffer, free of $MgCl_2$, $CaCl_2$, heparin, apyrase, and EDTA, and then incubated at 37°C for 45 min. In some experiments washed platelets were prepared by gel filtration (38). These platelets aggregated with 10^{-5}M ADP or 10^{-5}M epinephrine when 2 mg/ml human fibrinogen was added to the suspension. Collagen-induced aggregation did not require fibrinogen but was enhanced by its addition.

In Vitro Platelet Aggregation

Platelet aggregation was measured turbidometrically (20) with a Bio-Data aggregometer (Bio-Data Corp., Willow Grove, Pa.). In a typical experiment, 0.4 ml of PRP or washed platelets was warmed to 37°C for 3 min in a flat-bottomed cylindrical cuvette. The platelets were then stirred in the aggregometer at 1200 rpm, a baseline was obtained on the recorder, and 0.05 ml of PAM was added. Aggregation was recorded as an increase in light transmission, with PPP representing 100% transmission. In experiments

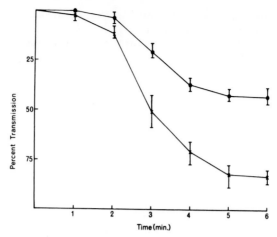

FIG. 1. Induction of rabbit platelet aggregation in heparinized PRP by 10⁷ intact 3T3 (●——●) or SV3T3 (x——x) cells. Each point (± S.E.M.) represents the average of four experiments.

where inhibitors of aggregation were assayed, 0.05 ml of inhibitor or 0.05 ml of Veronal buffer was followed by 0.05 ml of PAM.

Centrifugation of PAM

To determine whether PAM was sedimentable, 0.5 ml of extract was spun at 100,000 x g for 1 hr at 4°C in a Beckman L2-65B ultracentrifuge equipped with an SW40Ti rotor (Beckman Instruments, Inc., Fullerton, Calif.). Following centrifugation, the supernatant was removed, and the pellet was resuspended in 0.5 ml of Veronal buffer.

Lipid Analysis

For lipid identification, cells were labeled metabolically as follows. First, 44 μCi of ¹⁴C-oleic acid were evaporated in a test tube under N₂ and redissolved in 24 ml of E4 containing 10% fetal calf serum and 170 μl of 1% bovine serum albumin (BSA) (Miles Laboratories, Elkhart, Ind.). Six confluent (6 cm) dishes, each containing either SV3T3 or 3T3, received 2 ml of this medium and were incubated for 24 hr. Five dishes, each containing 3T3 or SV3T3, were extracted for PAM in the usual fashion with 1M urea and then extracted for total lipids. One dish each of 3T3 or SV3T3 was extracted for total lipids at room temperature as follows (2). Dishes were washed once with PBS, and cells were scraped into 2 ml of PBS with a rubber policeman. The cell suspension was placed in a tight-fitting Dounce homogenizer with a Teflon-coated pestle; 2.5 ml of chloroform and 5 ml of methanol were added, and the suspension was homogenized with 25 strokes.

Then 2.5 ml of chloroform were added, and the mixture was homogenized again with 25 strokes, followed by addition of 2.5 ml H_2O and an additional 25 strokes. The final homogenate was filtered through a scintered glass funnel, and the phases were allowed to separate in a glass tube for 10 min. The top aqueous phase was discarded, and the bottom nonpolar phase was dried and redissolved for thin-layer chromatography (TLC) on silica plates (Merck & Co., Rahway, N.J.) with a development buffer consisting of 65 parts chloroform, 25 parts methanol, 4 parts H_2O, and 1 part acetic acid.

The radioactive urea extract was dialyzed against H_2O, lyophilized, redissolved in 2 ml of PBS, and extracted with organic solvents in an identical manner to the cells. Total recovery of radioactivity was approximately 80% following TLC.

Enzyme Treatment of PAM

Ten microliters of an enzyme solution were added to 100 μl of PAM (100 μg/ml protein) to give the final enzyme concentration shown in Table IV, and the mixture was incubated for 1 hr at 37°C. Enzymes were shown to be active with their respective substrates prior to use. A 50 μl amount of either treated PAM, or enzyme alone diluted 1:11 in Veronal buffer, was used in the aggregation assay. No enzyme induced aggregation by itself, nor did enzyme treatment of platelets render them unresponsive to $2 \times 10^{-5}M$ ADP or to untreated PAM added simultaneously. To further ensure that the presence of enzyme was not making the platelets specifically unresponsive to PAM, treated PAM was centrifuged as previously described to pellet activity, and the pellet was resuspended in Veronal buffer prior to reacting with the platelets.

Phospholipase-A_2 was boiled for 10 min prior to use in order to inactivate possible contaminants. Neuraminidase treatment was performed in the presence of 2 mM phenylmethyl sulfonyl fluoride (PMSF) to inhibit any contaminating protease activity.

Quantitation of the Release with ^{14}C-serotonin

Serotonin release was determined essentially as described (10). Briefly, 50 μCi of ^{14}C-serotonin were dissolved in 6.75 ml of 70% ethanol, and 5 μl were added to 5 ml of PRP. The mixture was incubated for 15 min at 37°C. ^{14}C-serotonin uptake was measured by subtracting free radioactivity in the supernatant from the total radioactivity obtained following sonication of the platelets. Release of ^{14}C-serotonin from the platelets was quantified by stirring 0.4 ml of labeled platelets in the aggregometer with 50 μl of $2 \times 10^{-5}M$ ADP, 50 μl of Veronal buffer, or 50 μl of PAM. Following aggregation, platelets or aggregates were pelleted by centrifugation at 2000 x g for 15 min at room temperature, and 100 μl of the supernatant were assayed for radioactivity in 5 ml of Aquasol in a liquid scintillation counter. Percent release was calculated as radioactivity in the PAM-containing supernatant

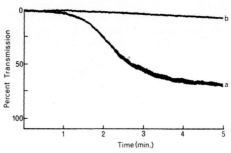

FIG 2. Induction of rabbit platelet aggregation in heparinized PRP by 10^6 intact SV3T3 cells before (a) and following (b) treatment of monolayer cells with 0.25 ml of 0.25% trypsin for 5 min at 37°C. Trypsin was neutralized with 0.5 ml of 0.25% soybean trypsin inhibitor prior to the preparation of the cell suspension for the aggregation assay. Then 0.05 ml of cells was added to 0.4 ml of PRP. Data taken from one of five experiments with similar results.

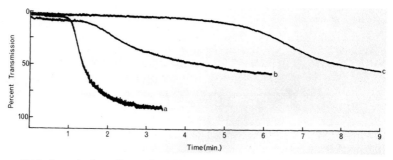

FIG 3. Induction of rabbit platelet aggregation in heparinized PRP by 1M urea extracts from SV3T3 cells at a final protein concentration of (a) 40 μg/ml or (b) 2 μg/ml and from 3T3 cells (c) at 40 μg/ml. Data taken from one of 20 experiments with similar results.

minus background radioactivity (either ADP or buffer) divided by total radioactivity taken up by the platelet suspension.

Chemicals, Enzymes, and Reagents

All chemicals were reagent grade. Enzymes were obtained from the following companies: apyrase, β-galactosidase (grade IV), phospholipase-A (bee venom), and neuraminidase (type V) were obtained from Sigma Chemical Co., St. Louis, Mo.; trypsin, treated with tosyl phenyl chloroketone (TPCK), and soybean trypsin inhibitor were obtained from Worthington Biochemical Corp., Freehold, N.J.; NP-40 was obtained from Particle Data, Inc., Elmhurst, Ill.;

and Tween 80 from Sigma. Epinephrine hydrochloride was obtained
from Parke-Davis & Co., Detroit, Mich. Purified fibrinogen was a
gift of Dr. Alan Johnson, New York University Medical Center.
Connective tissue collagen was prepared and employed as described
previously (43). ^{14}C-serotonin, 30 mCi/mM, was obtained from
Amersham/Searle Corp., Arlington Heights, Ill. ^{14}C-oleic acid,
55.7 mCi/mM, and Aquasol were obtained from New England Nuclear,
Boston, Mass.

RESULTS

Whole Cells

   Intact SV3T3 transformed cells were capable of inducing platelet aggregation after a lag period of 1 to 2 min (Fig. 1). When
50 μl of transformed cells at an initial concentration of 10^7
cells/ml were added to 0.4 ml of PRP, the final maximal level of
aggregation (optical density change) reached was 80% of that
achieved by the addition of 2 x 10^{-5}M ADP. The normal 3T3 line
was also capable of inducing moderate aggregation following a
slightly longer lag period than that observed with the transformed
cell. However, the final percentage of aggregation induced by
the normal cell line was approximately 40% of the ADP control
(Fig. 1). Treatment of a monolayer of intact SV3T3 cells with 2.5
mg/ml trypsin completely abolished its ability to aggregate platelets (Fig. 2).

Urea Extract

   A urea extract of SV3T3 cells induced platelet aggregation at
a final concentration of 40 μg/ml protein (Fig. 3). In contrast,
medium conditioned by the same cell type for an identical length
of time required approximately fivefold to 10-fold higher concentration of protein to induce a similar degree of aggregation
(data not shown). Dilution of the extracted SV3T3 cell line PAM
by a factor of 20 (from 40 to 2 μg/ml) resulted in a loss of activity (Fig. 3), demonstrating the sensitivity of the system to
dilution. Normal 3T3 cell extracts, at 40 μg/ml, were capable of
inducing only slight aggregation after a prolonged lag period
(Fig. 3).
   The transformed cell extract was more effective in heparin-PRP,
as were the intact cells, in agreement with the results of
others (10).

Inhibitors of PAM

   As shown in Table I, several compounds which inhibit the secondary wave of platelet aggregation (41) also prevented PAM induction of platelet aggregation. Thus 5 mM EDTA, 0.05 mM indomethacin, 0.1 mM adenosine, and 0.1 mM N6,02^{1}-dibutyrl cyclic AMP
all inhibited PAM activity.

TABLE I.   Inhibition of PAM-induced aggregation with inhibitors
of the platelet release reaction[a]

Inhibitor	Aggregating Agent	Percent Aggregation
Veronal buffer	PAM	100
Veronal buffer	2×10^{-5}M ADP	100
5 mM EDTA	PAM	0
0.1 mM dBcAMP[b]	PAM	1-30
0.1 mM dBcAMP	2×10^{-5}M ADP	0
0.1 mM adenosine	PAM	0
0.1 mM adenosine	2×10^{-5}M ADP	0
0.05 mM indomethacin	PAM	10

[a]All inhibitors were incubated with heparinized rabbit PRP for
6-9 min at 37°C prior to the addition of PAM, 10 μg/ml. Inhibitor concentration is that achieved following dilution of the inhibitor in PRP. Each experiment was performed 3 or more times.
dBcAMP = $N^6,0^{2'}$-dibutyrl cyclic AMP.

TABLE II.   Release of ^{14}C-serotonin following addition of PAM
to heparinized rabbit PRP[a]

Addition	CPM in supernatant	Percent Release
Veronal buffer	399	2
2×10^{-5}M ADP	387	2
PAM	10,255	53
Sonication	19,350	100

[a]Percent release was calculated as radioactivity in PAM-containing supernatant minus background radioactivity (buffer)
divided by total radioactivity taken up by the platelet suspension. Results are an average of 2 determinations.

Release of ^{14}C-serotonin

Direct measurement of the release reaction was performed by
quantitating ^{14}C-serotonin release from aggregated platelets.
The results, shown in Table II, indicate that PAM accomplishes
irreversible aggregation by inducing platelet release.

Non-inhibitors of PAM

Certain proteases induce platelet aggregation (3), and tumor
cells frequently synthesize higher levels of proteases than do
their normal counterparts (12,28). Therefore, an attempt was made
to inhibit PAM with several specific protease inhibitors known to

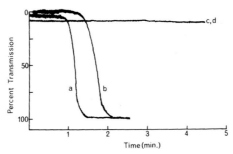

FIG. 4. Platelet aggregation following sedimentation
of PAM by ultracentrifugation. a, Original SV3T3 extract;
b, resuspended extract pellet in original volume of Veronal buffer following centrifugation at 100,000 x g for
1 hr; c, supernatant following centrifugation; and d,
3T3 extract pellet following centrifugation and resuspen-
sion of pellet in Veronal buffer. The difference in lag
period between a and b is not significant.

TABLE III.   Effect of protease inhibitors on PAM-mediated
platelet aggregation[a]

Inhibitor	Final Concentration	% Aggregation
Veronal buffer	--	100
EACA (Epsilon-amino-caproic acid)	0.8 mM	95
Soybean trypsin inhibitor	50-500 μg/ml	98
Trasylol	50 U/ml	95
PMSF	2 mM	90
DFP (diisopropylfluoro-phosphate)	2.5 mM	82

[a]Percent release was calculated as radioactivity in PAM-
containing supernatant minus background radioactivity (buffer)
divided by total radioactivity taken up by the platelet suspension. Results are an average of 2 determinations.

interfere with transformed cell plasminogen activation (18). All
inhibitors were assayed for activity on appropriate substrates
prior to use. For example, 2.5 mM DFP inhibited thrombin-induced
platelet aggregation at a concentration of 0.1 μg/ml. The results
given in Table III clearly indicate that PAM activity is not related to any increase in proteolytic activity associated with
transformed cell plasma membranes. Thus EACA (0.8 mM), soybean
trypsin inhibitor (50-500 μg/ml), trasylol (50 units/ml), PMSF
(2 mM), and DFP (2.5 mM) had no significant effect on platelet

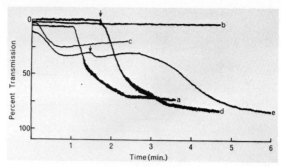

FIG. 5. Synergistic effect of PAM and epinephrine on platelet aggregation in rabbit PRP. a, 10 μg/ml PAM; b, 1 μg/ml PAM; c, 10^{-5}M epinephrine; d, 1 μg/ml PAM followed by 10^{-5}M epinephrine; e, 10^{-5}M epinephrine followed by 1 μg/ml PAM. Concentrations given are those achieved following dilution of the material in PRP during the assay. Initial additions were done at time zero. Second additions (in d and e) are indicated by arrows. Data taken from one of four experiments with similar results.

TABLE IV.   <u>Effect of boiling, enzymes, non-ionic detergents, and sonication on PAM activity[a]</u>

Treatment	Final Concentration or Time	Percent Aggregation	N[b]
Boiling	15 min	0	3
Boiling and storage at 0°C for 2 weeks	--	30-40	2
Trypsin-TPCK	1 mg/ml	0	5
Neuraminidase	2 mg/ml	0	5
Phospholipase-A_2	0.1 μg/ml	0	5
NP-40	0.1%	0	3
Tween-80	0.1%	0	3
Sonication	15 sec	0	2
β-Galactosidase	0.5 mg/ml	83	2

[a]All enzymes, in 10 μl volume, were incubated with 100 μl of PAM, 100 μg/ml, for 1 hr at 37°C. PAM was then sedimented at 100,000 x g for 1 hr at 4°C, and the pellet was resuspended in 100 μl of Veronal buffer. Of this material, 50 μl were used for platelet-aggregation studies with heparinized rabbit PRP.
[b]N = number of experiments

aggregation.

Centrifugation of PAM

The urea-extracted PAM from SV3T3 cells can be pelleted by centrifugation at 100,000 x g for 1 hr at $4°C$. The results shown in Fig. 4 clearly demonstrate that all the activity was recoverable in the pellet, with no residual PAM remaining in the supernatant. The ability to pellet the material provided a means of removing enzyme from the enzyme-treated PAM in order to discriminate between the effect of enzyme on PAM and on the platelet surface.

Effect of Boiling, Enzymes, Non-ionic Detergents, or Sonication on PAM and PRP

The following treatments, listed in Table IV, completely destroyed PAM activity: 1) boiling for 15 min (partial activity could be restored, following boiling, by storage for several weeks at $4°C$); 2) crystalline trypsin at 1 mg/ml; 3) neuraminidase at 2 mg/ml in the presence of 2 mM PMSF; 4) boiled phospholipase-A_2 at 0.1 μg/ml; 5) non-ionic detergents, NP-40 (0.1%) and Tween-80 (0.1%); 6) sonication for 15 sec at $0°C$.

β-Galactosidase at 5 mg/ml had no effect on PAM.

PAM was washed by centrifugation and resuspended in fresh buffer prior to mixing with platelets in order to ensure that these enzymes or compounds did not affect platelets directly, making them unresponsive to PAM. Furthermore, platelet aggregation could be induced by addition of fresh PAM to PRP containing inactivated PAM. Therefore the effect was on PAM directly, not on platelet receptors for PAM.

Lipid Analysis of PAM

Extracted lipids, labeled with ^{14}C-oleic acid for 24 hr, were analyzed by TLC followed by scintillation counting of areas corresponding to specific lipid components. Preliminary experiments revealed that a steady-state level of incorporation had been achieved by this time. Therefore differences between the normal and transformed cells probably reflect differences in composition. This hypothesis is supported by a comparison of the radioactivity recovered from intact 3T3 and SV3T3 cells (Table V), wherein similar percentages of radioactivity were found for all phospholipid types identified. The results shown in Table V indicate that the SV3T3 extract, when compared to the 3T3 extract, incorporated 1.8-fold more radioactivity into phospholipid (63% vs. 36%), 1.9-fold more radioactivity into PS/PI (41% vs. 21%), and 0.6-fold less radioactivity into sphingomyelin (15% vs. 6%).

TABLE V. Incorporation of C-oleic acid into phospholipid fractions of cells and urea extracts from normal 3T3 and transformed SV3T3 cells.

| Phospholipids: | CPM recovered following TLC | | | |
| | 3T3 | | SV3T3 | |
	Cells (%)	Extract (%)	Cells (%)	Extract (%)
SM	764 (5.8%)[a]	200 (14.9%)	207 (3.0%)	135 (5.8%)
PC	9168 (69.5)	624 (46.4)	4407 (63.4)	801 (34.5)
PS/PI	1094 (8.3)	287 (21.3)	508 (7.3)	940 (40.5)
PE	2162 (16.4)	235 (17.5)	1832 (26.3)	446 (19.2)
Total	13,188	1346	6954	2322
Total lipid[b]	16,779	3733	14,148	3680
% phospholipid[c]		36%		63%

SM = sphingomyelin; PC = phosphatidylcholine; PE = phosphatidylethanolamine.
Results are an average of 2 determinations which gave nearly identical results.

[a] % calculated as $\dfrac{\text{cpm in individual phospholipid}}{\text{total phospholipid cpm}} \times 100.$

[b] Total recoverable cpm following TLC

[c] % calculated as $\dfrac{\text{cpm in total phospholipid}}{\text{total lipid cpm}} \times 100.$

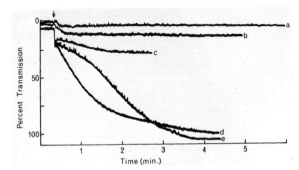

FIG. 6.   Effect of ADP, fibrinogen, and PAM on the aggregation of washed human platelets. Addition of PAM
(10 μg/ml) in the a, absence of b, precence or fibrinogen. Addition of ADP (2 x 10^{-5}M) in the c, absence or
d, presence of fibringoen (2 mg/ml) or e, PAM. Initial
incubations were started at time zero, and additions
were made when indicated by arrow. Data taken from one
of seven experiments with similar results.

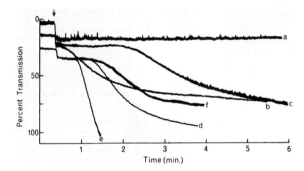

FIG. 7.   Effect of epinephrine, collagen, fibrinogen,
and PAM on the aggregation of washed human platelets.
Addition of epinephrine (10^{-5}M) in the a, absence or
b, presence of fibrinogen or c, PAM. Addition of
collagen (1:3200 dilution) in the d, absence or e,
presence of fibrinogen or f, PAM. Initial incubations
were started at time zero, and additions were made when
indicated by arrow. Data taken from one of four
experiments with similar results.

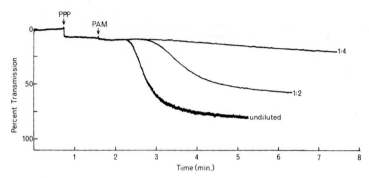

FIG. 8. Aggregation of gel-filtered platelets in the presence of PPP and PAM. The addition of 50 μl of PPP (arrow) to 0.4 ml of gel-filtered platelets prior to the addition of 50 μl of PAM (arrow) reconstituted the aggregation-promoting activity of PAM. Dilution of PPP (1:2 and 1:4) with Veronal buffer resulted in a concentration-dependent loss of reconstituting activity. Data taken from one of three experiments with similar results.

PAM Synergism in Rabbit PRP

Dilutions of PAM were prepared which were below the threshold concentration required for platelet aggregation. Epinephrine, ADP, and collagen were also diluted to levels which were incapable of promoting platelet aggregation. By mixing these subthreshold concentrations of aggregating agents with dilute PAM (Fig. 5), we could demonstrate a synergistic effect between PAM and epinephrine at 1 μg/ml and 10^{-5}M, respectively, regardless of the order of addition. Neither ADP nor collagen proved to be synergistic with PAM when assayed in rabbit PRP (data not shown).

Effect of PAM on Washed Platelets

PAM did not aggregate washed platelets in the presence or absence of fibrinogen (a and b, Fig. 6) in most experiments (a small optical density change of 10% to 15% was occasionally noted in the presence of fibrinogen plus PAM). However, the washed human platelet system developed was responsive to platelet aggregation induced by ADP (c and d, Fig. 6) or epinephrine (a and b, Fig. 7) in the presence of purified human fibrinogen and to collagen (d and e, Fig. 7) in the absence or presence of fibrinogen. Of particular interest was the observation that PAM could replace the fibrinogen requirement for ADP-induced aggregation (e, Fig. 6) or epinephrine-induced aggregation (c, Fig. 7) but not for collagen-induced aggregation (f, Fig. 7).

We have also observed that preincubation of PPP with gel-filtered (washed) platelets, prior to the addition of PAM, restores PAM's ability to induce platelet aggregation (Fig. 8). This was concentration-dependent. However, when boiled PPP was employed, no restoration of activity was observed (data not shown).

Further studies on the plasma factor have revealed the following, (the details of which will be published elsewhere): 1) Incubation of PAM with plasma (1:1) at 37°C for 10 minutes, produces
an 'activated PAM' which abolishes the 1-2 minute lag period
noted in the absence of prior incubation; 2) Heating of this
'activated PAM' at 56°C for 30 minutes does not destroy PAM activity, whereas heating of plasma at 56°C for 30 minutes does destroy its ability to support PAM-induced aggregation; 3) 'Activated PAM' loses its ability to aggregate washed platelets if it is
separated from plasma by centrifugation at 100,000 g for 1 hour
and the plasma supernatant is removed. However, readdition of
fresh plasma, or plasma heated to 56°C for 30 minutes restores
the activity.

Thus, a heat labile factor is required to activate PAM and
abolish the lag period and a heat stable factor is required for
the 'activated PAM' to be operative. Preliminary studies indicate that the heat labile factor is complement, since treatment
of plasma with cobra venom abolishes its ability to activate PAM.
Since C-4 deficient plasma retains the ability to activate PAM,
it appears that the alternative complement pathway is involved.
The requirement of complement for tumor cell-induced platelet
aggregation has recently been reported by Gasic et al at this
Symposium.

DISCUSSION

In agreement with Gasic and co-workers (5-7,10), we have demonstrated that viral transformants of established cell lines will
cause platelet aggregation whereas the normal parental line is
much less effective (Fig. 1). Indeed, it is conceivable that the
low activity of the nontransformed cells could represent initial
signs of spontaneous in vitro cell transformation. In addition,
1M urea extraction of plasma membrane components from the transformed cells permits this effect to be demonstrated by cell-free
extracts (Fig. 3). The extraction of normal cells yields considerably less biologically active PAM. It is of interest that although the intact normal cells contained one-half the platelet-
aggregating activity of transformed cells, the urea extract of
the normal cells contained 20-fold less PAM.

Both transformed cells and their cell-free extracts cause
platelets in PRP to aggregate in a similar fashion: a lag period
of 1 to 3 minutes followed by rapid platelet aggregation accompanied by the release reaction. The sensitivity of the tumor
cell and the cell-free extract to trypsin was also similar. It
is therefore likely that platelet aggregation induced by intact
cells and extract is promoted by equivalent factors. PAM operates
via the release reaction and requires divalent cation, since
inhibitors of the secondary wave of platelet aggregation abolish
PAM-induced aggregation of PRP (Table I). PAM operates best in
heparin-PRP rather than citrate-PRP and does not operate in the

presence of EDTA (Table 1).

The mechanism of action of PAM-induced aggregation is unique because PAM aggregates PRP but does not aggregate washed platelets, which are capable of being aggregated by ADP or epinephrine in the presence of fibrinogen or by collagen in the absence of fibrinogen. However, PAM, like fibrinogen, does support ADP- and epinephrine-induced platelet aggregation and may operate via a mechanism similar to that of fibrinogen in the washed platelet system. It is conceivable that PAM has two activities or sites: one which aggregates platelets in PRP (requiring a plasma factor) and another which supports washed platelet aggregation in the absence of fibrinogen.

The plasma requirement is of interest. A heat labile factor (probably alternative pathway complement components) is necessary for the activation of PAM and the elimination of the lag period. A heat stable factor is required for activated PAM to be operative.

Gasic et al (10) have classified the interaction of platelets in PRP and tumor cells into three stages depending on the percent of platelet aggregation and the release of serotonin. By these criteria, SV3T3 and PAM are equivalent to type III tumor cells, since platelet aggregation was generally greater than 80% (Figs. 1 and 3) and serotonin release was measured at 53% (Table II).

Many transformed cells have been shown to have increased levels of proteolytic enzymes (12,40) including the transformed lines used in these studies (33). Since platelets are sensitive to aggregation by specific proteases (3,27), we attempted to inhibit PAM-induced aggregation by protease inhibitors known to prevent plasminogen activation by these tumor cells (EACA and soybean trypsin inhibitor) as well as additional protease inhibitors. As shown in Table III, none of these inhibitors prevented platelet aggregation with PAM. This finding is in agreement with a report (10) which showed no correlation between the ability of tumor cells to induce platelet aggregation and their fibrinolytic activity in vitro.

We have demonstrated that PAM is a complex mixture of protein, lipid, and carbohydrate assembled in a macromolecular form capable of sedimentation at 100,000 x g for 1 hour. Destruction of PAM activity by trypsin, neuraminidase, or phospholipase-A_2 indicates that several components interact to produce PAM activity. This interaction may involve maintenance of a vesicular configuration, since sonication will also reduce PAM activity. Attempts to replace lipid by neutral detergents and maintain activity have been unsuccessful, and it appears that the lipid moiety may play more than a simple structural role in promoting platelet aggregation. This would be compatible with the previously demonstrated ability of free fatty acids to cause platelet aggregation (17) in the presence of heparin and calcium ions. Sodium salts of free fatty acids dissolved in lecithin cause platelet aggregation in PRP (21), and low concentrations of stearic acid enhance epinephrine-induced platelet aggregation (1), an effect also observed with PAM (Fig. 5). Thrombofax, a poorly characterized commercially

prepared cephalin, will also cause platelet aggregation following
a lag period (4). This aggregation is accompanied by ^{14}C-seroton-
in release. To our knowledge, the effect of purified phospholipids on platelet aggregation has not been tested. However, phos-
pholipid-containing liposomes will fuse with and cause fusion of
several different cell types (24,29,30). It is conceivable that
platelets may aggregate in their presence. Indeed, PS is speci-
ally active in promoting fusion (25,31) and is a lipid constitu-
ent probably increased in concentration in SV3T3 extracts (Table
V).

The involvement of sialic acid is interesting in light of a
report demonstrating increased levels of sialic acid-containing
glycolipids in serum samples obtained from mice bearing transplantable mammary carcinomas, compared to normal animals (22).
The sialic acid components were shown to be present in the gangli-
osides. The sensitivity of PAM to neuraminidase but not to β-
galactosidase indicates that PAM and the material present in the
serum of tumor-bearing animals may be related. An antibody currently being prepared against PAM may help to resolve this
question.

The ability to sediment PAM activity by centrifugation implies
a large particle size for the material. This led us to attempt
to increase PAM yield by treatment of intact cells with formalde-
hyde, a procedure reported to increase vesicle formation in SV3T3
cells (36). Although we have confirmed this observation, no PAM
activity could be recovered in the cell-free supernatants of our
formaldehyde-treated tumor cell lines. In addition, treatment of
PAM with trypsin, neuraminidase, or phospholipase-A_2 still allowed
recovery of sedimentable material following centrifugation, indicating the presence of macromolecular components, despite complete
loss of aggregating activity. We therefore suggest that both the
chemical constituents of PAM and the physical nature of the material are relevant to its in vitro platelet-aggregating activity.

Extraction of intact cells with 1M urea also leads to an en-
richment of a normal cell plasma membrane component (42) desig-
nated CAF (32). Since transformed cells lack this glycoprotein
(35), it was possible that PAM activity of normal cells was inhibited by the presence of CAF. We therefore assayed PAM activity
following addition of exogenous CAF at 50 μg/ml and found that
CAF has no inhibitory or synergistic activity with PAM. CAF alone
at 50 μg/ml, also has no effect on platelet aggregation in PRP
(data not shown).

Since fibroblasts synthesize collagen and collagen can induce
platelet aggregation in vitro (43), it was necessary to determine
whether PAM activity may be related to this protein. Such does
not appear to be the case because 1) treatment of tumor cells
with collagenase does not interfere with their aggregation-promoting activity (6), 2) PAM and collagen are not additive in
inducing platelet aggregation, 3) transformation leads to a decrease in collagen biosynthesis (13), and 4) collagen is capable
of aggregating washed platelets (d and e, Fig. 7) but PAM is not
(a and b, Fig. 6).

We therefore conclude that tumor cells contain a urea-extractable sedimentable particle which is capable of aggregating platelets via the release reaction in the presence of a plasma factor and divalent cation. Its mechanism of action may be related to its ability to replace fibrinogen as a supporting medium for washed platelet aggregation with ADP or epinephrine. PAM is heat-sensitive and requires intact sialic acid, phospholipid, and trypsin-sensitive protein constituents for activity. The particle is denatured by non-ionic detergents and sonication, suggesting that lipid-particle configuration may also play a role in its activity.

REFERENCES

1. Ardlie, N.G., Kinlough, R.L., Glew, G., and Schwartz, C.J. (1966): Aust. J. Exp. Biol. Med. Sci., 44:105.
2. Bligh, E.B., and Dyer, W.J. (1959): Can. J. Biochem. Physiol. 37:911.
3. Davey, M.G., and Luscher, E.F. (1966): Thromb. Diath. Haemorrh., 20 (Suppl.):283.
4. DeClerck, F., Borgers, M., Vermylen, J., and DeGaetano, G. (1974): Scand. J. Haematol., 12:90.
5. Gasic, G.J., Boettiger, D., Catalfamo, J.L., Gasic, T.B., and Stewart, G.J. (1978): Cancer Res., 38:2950.
6. Gasic, G.J., Gasic, T.B., Galanti, N., Johnson, T., and Murphy, S. (1973): Int. J. Cancer, 11:704.
7. Gasic, G.J., Gasic, T.B., and Jimenez, S.A. (1977): Thromb. Res., 10:33.
8. Gasic, G.J., Gasic, T.B., and Murphy, S. (1972): Lancet, 2:932.
9. Gasic. G.J.. Gasic, T.B., and Stewart, C.C. (1968): Proc. Natl. Acad. Sci. USA, 61:46
10. Gasic, G.J., Koch, P.A.G., Hsu, B., Gasic, T.B., and Niewiarowski, S. (1976): Z. Krebsforsch, 86:263.
11. Gastpar, H. (1977): J. Med., 8:103.
12. Goldberg, A.R. (1974): Cell, 2:95.
13. Green, H., Goldberg, B., and Todaro, G.J. (1966): Nature, 212:631.
14. Hagmar, B., and Boeryd, B. (1969): Pathol. Eur., 4:274.
15. Hilgard, P. (1973): Br. J. Cancer, 28:429.
16. Hilgard, P., and Gordon-Smith, E.C. (1974): Br. J. Haematol., 26:651.
17. Hoak, J.C., Warner, E.D., and Connor, W.E. (1967): Circ. Res. 20:11.
18. Hynes, R.O., and Pearlstein, E. (1976): J. Supramolec. Struct., 4:1.
19. Jones, D.S., Wallace, A.C., and Fraser, E.F. (1971): J. Natl. Cancer Inst., 46:493.
20. Karpatkin, S. (1978): Blood, 51:307.
21. Kerr, J.W., Pirrie, R., MacAulay, I., and Bronte-Stewart, B. (1965): Lancet, 1:1296.

22. Kloppel, T.M., Keenan, T.W., Freeman, M.J., and Morre, D.J. (1977): Proc. Natl. Acad. Sci. USA, 74:3011.
23. Kramer, P.M. (1968): Biochim. Biophys. Acta, 167:205.
24. Martin, F., and MacDonald, R. (1974): Nature, 252:161.
25. Miller, C., and Racker, E. (1976): J. Membr. Biol., 26:319.
26. Mustard, J.F., Perry, D.W., Ardlie, N.G., and Packham, M.A. (1972): Br. J. Haematol., 22:193.
27. Niewiarowski, S., Senyi, A.F., and Gilles, P. (1973): J. Clin. Invest., 52:1647.
28. Ossowski, L., Unkeless, J.C., Tobia, A., Quigley, J.P., Rifkin, D.B., and Reich, E. (1973): J. Exp. Med., 137:112.
29. Pagano, R.E., Huang, L., and Wey, C. (1974): Nature, 252:166.
30. Papahadjopoulos, D., Mayhew, E., Poste, G., Smith, S., and Vail, W.J. (1974): Nature, 252:166.
31. Papahadjopoulos, D., Poste, G., Schaeffer, B.E., and Vail, W.J. (1974): Biochim. Biophys. Acta., 352:10.
32. Pearlstein, E. (1976): Nature, 262:497.
33. Pearlstein, E., Hynes, R.O., Franks, L.M., and Hemmings, V.J. (1976): Cancer Res., 36:1475.
34. Pearlstein, E., and Seaver, J. (1976): Biochim. Biophys. Acta, 426:589.
35. Pearlstein, E., and Waterfield, M.W. (1974): Biochim. Biophys. Acta, 362:1.
36. Scott, R.E. (1976): Science, 194:743.
37. Sindelar, W.F., Tralke, T.S., and Ketcham, A.S. (1975): J. Surg. Res., 18:137.
38. Tangen, D., and Berman, H.J. (1972): Adv. Exp. Med. Biol., 34:235.
39. Warren, B.A. (1973): J. Med., 4:150.
40. Warren, B.A. and Vales, O. (1972): Br. J. Exp. Pathol., 53:301.
41. Weiss, H.J. (1975): N. Engl. J. Med., 293:531.
42. Yamada, K.M., Yamada, S.S., and Pastan, I. (1975): Proc. Natl. Acad. Sci. USA, 72:3158.
43. Zucker, M.B., and Borelli, J. (1962): Proc. Soc. Exp. Biol. Med., 109:779.

Malignancy and the Hemostatic System,
edited by M. B. Donati et al.
Raven Press, New York © 1981.

Cancer Cell Procoagulant Activity

H. R. Gralnick

*Hematology Service, Clinical Pathology Department, Clinical Center,
National Institutes of Health, Bethesda, Maryland 20205*

Understanding the malignant cell in neoplastic processes has proven to be one of the cornerstones for the development of effective chemotherapy in malignant disease. Recently, the study of the coagulation and fibrinolytic potential of neoplastic cells has revealed that many different types of human tumors exhibit procoagulant or fibrinolytic activity far greater than that of comparable normal cells. From both experimental and clinical studies, it is clear that the coagulation system may play an important role in malignant tumors by promoting tumor growth by potentiating metastasis or by forming a protective environment to exclude chemotherapy from reaching the tumor. Thus, a greater understanding of the role of the cancer cell in coagulation could potentially lead to more effective therapy in the underlying tumor as well as adjuvant therapy to inhibit metastasis. Recent studies have suggested that the use of anticoagulation or anti-platelet drugs in certain types of tumors in conjunction with chemotherapy have resulted in increased numbers of responses. However, these studies are still far from complete and conflicting data exist.

O'Meara and coworkers (1-3) first described a cancer coagulative factor, although the specific type of procoagulant was never clearly defined. However, it was one of the initial studies which directed attention to the postulate that fibrin was regularly laid down around cancer cells invading tissue and that tumors contained materials which might be active in blood coagu-. lation, thus enhancing their ability to form fibrin and to invade surrounding tissue. Since then, many studies have examined the procoagulant activity of tumor cells. There have been several studies which have defined a tumor related procoagulant activity which is indistinguishable from tissue factor. Particularly rich sources have been in promyelocytes in acute promyelocytic leukemia (4-6), other forms of leukemia (7), mucus-secreting adenocarcinoma (8,9), gastric adenocarcinoma (10) and to a lesser degree in other carcinomas. The tissue factor is defined, in part, by the fact that it requires calcium and intact factor VII to activate factor X. The final expression of its activity involves the enzymatic conversion of prothrombin to thrombin by

57

factor Xa in the presence of calcium, factor V and phospholipid.
Then thrombin converts fibrinogen to fibrin. Other studies have
revealed different procoagulants which appear to be enzymes which
can directly convert factor X from its inactive state to its
activated state: Gordon and coworkers (11) as well as others
(12-13) demonstrated a direct factor X-activating activity in a
cancer extract. Dr. Semeraro will discuss these types of procoagulants in the accompanying paper. It is clear, though, that
this factor does not require the presence of factor VII to express
its biologic activity. Other factor X-activating enzymes have
been described, however, whether these all represent one class of
specific tumor-related enzymes is not clear from the data pre-
sently available.

Although not a procoagulant enzyme, increased fibrin cross-
linking or transglutaminase activities have been described in
experimental tumors compared to normal tissue (14). In particular, there have been suggestions that in several mouse tumors the
involvement of transglutaminase is very important in tumor growth
and metastases. Studies of various tumors in mice reveal that
there is an inverse correlation between the transglutaminase level
in a given strain of animal and the average survival time (15),
while studies in human breast cancer and melanoma show a correlation between frequency of metastasis and transglutaminase content
(16). The exact mechanism of how the transglutaminase interacts
with tumors is not clear. It has been suggested that there is
some correlation between transglutaminase activity and the ability
of the tumor to penetrate normal tissue.

As you will read in other articles in this book, it is clear
that tumors have interactions with platelets which in some way
may promoted the spread or growth of the tumor. It is not clear
whether these are all physical interactions between tumor cells
and platelets or whether tumor cells are able to recruit platelets
by release of mediators from the tumor cell which results in
platelet accumulation at or near the tumor cell.

Our interest in cancer cell procoagulant activity was initiated by the almost invariable occurrence of the syndrome of intravascular coagulation with the disease hypergranular promyelocytic
leukemia (APL) (17-20). Previously, Quigley (4) had demonstrated
that the white cells from patients with APL could act like
thromboplastin when incubated with normal plasma, and suggested
that there was a clot-promoting activity present in these white
cells. Subsequent studies by us and others have revealed that,
indeed, cells of APL have increased amounts of the procoagulant
which fits the definition of tissue factor. Extracts from these
cells could correct the clotting defects in factor XII, XI, VIII,
IX and V deficient plasma but had no effect on factor VII or X
deficient plasma. In addition, utilizing a two-stage technique
to measure the tissue factor, it was found that these cells contained large amounts of tissue factor when compared to normal
mature granulocytes. The tissue factor isolated from APL cells
cross reacts immunologically with human brain thromboplastin (21).

Subsequent studies with myeloblasts from patients with acute myelogenous leukemia (AML) and lymphoblasts from patients with acute lymphoblastic leukemia (ALL) revealed that the large amount of tissue factor activity of the promyelocytes was not a finding present in all hematopoietic tumor cells, but appeared to be unique only for the promyelocytes, since both the myeloblasts and the lymphoblasts had lesser amounts of tissue factor activity per cell and per mg of protein than did the normal mature granulocyte. Further studies of the cells' fibrinolytic activity revealed that some of the promyelocytes in APL also had increased fibrinolytic and/or proteolytic activity as measured by lysis on fibrin plates, hydrolysis of casein or proteolysis of denatured hemoglobin. Again, the cells in AML and ALL were not found to have any significant increase in their fibrinolytic activity.

When one compared the findings of the in-vitro assays of coagulation and the procoagulant activity with the clinical findings in APL, it was clear that there was a very good correlation between the level of tissue factor activity and the hemorrhagic syndromes associated with these three types of leukemia. We have studied the cells of seven patients with APL and have found all to have increased levels of tissue factor activity, while three of seven patients had increased levels of fibrinolytic activity. In all seven patients there has been a marked hemorrhagic syndrome associated with their acute leukemia.

Early in the course of our studies, we realized both from our own work and that of other laboratories, that the most likely cause of hemorrhagic diathesis in APL was intravascular coagulation. Subsequently, we have treated 15 patients with heparin from the time of diagnosis of their disease rather than waiting for excessive bleeding to occur. We attempt to anticoagulate the individual once the diagnosis of APL has been confirmed, platelet support has been started and before chemotherapy is initiated. To date, we have lost only one patient due to hemorrhage or thrombosis; this individual had a platelet count of less than 1,000/μl for over 24 hours. The patient died of intracerebral hemorrhage, in part related to thrombocytopenia, intravascular coagulation and anticoagulation.

A recent study has shown that a group of patients with APL who received heparin had a greater overall survival rate than another group of patients who did not receive any heparin (22). Thus, the data at the present time appear to suggest that heparin is beneficial in the treatment of the acute phase of APL. However, other authors have stressed that heparin may be of limited value while others have indicated that the coagulopathy of their patients is really not intravascular coagulation.

Experimental studies have indicated that anticoagulation may have a beneficial effect in the arrest of tumor growth (a direct cytotoxic effect), in inhibiting metastases and in enhancing the tissue distribution and clearance of certain chemotherapeutic agents. It is clear in experimental studies that the use of heparin or coumadin has been shown to inhibit thromboplastin generation and thrombin formation and to have some effect on normal as well as neoplastic cell by inhibiting migration, decreasing growth potential and attachment to endothelium. All of these may play a significant role in any potential anti-tumor effect in addition to the anticoagulant effect itself. However, recent studies suggest that anticoagulants have no direct cytotoxic effect (23). One thing that appears to be clear is that in experimental tumors, both heparin and warfarin anticoagulation have been shown to decrease the incidence of metastases, primarily pulmonary or hepatic metastases, when tumor cells are injected into the vena cava. But, this decrease in metastases only occurs when the number of tumor cells injected is less than 10^5. When 10^5 or 10^6 cells are injected, pulmonary metastases are increased by anticoagulation (24). Long-term warfarin therapy of tumor-bearing animals causes a decrease in metastasis formation, and in animals with transplanted sarcomas, coumadin anticoagulant decreased the incidence of pulmonary metastases and increased the survival in animals following amputation of the primary tumor (24).

Thus, following the experimental studies of mice with transplanted sarcomas, my coworkers and I embarked on a study of preoperative and post-operative anticoagulation with coumadin for patients undergoing amputation of extremities for osteosarcomas. In this study, we have found that the patients who had adequate pre-operative anticoagulation had an increased 5-year survival regardless of the site of their tumor. In fact, of 9 patients who were fully studied, 5 (56%) are alive with no evidence of disease 5-8 years after the surgical procedure. In addition, the overall survival for the anticoagulated patients versus an historic control of non-anticoagulated patients revealed a marked difference in the percent survival for 2 years or more, 70% versus 20% and for 4 years, 60% versus 17% (25).

The complications of anticoagulation are primarily a slight increase in operative blood loss and an increase in post-operative bleeding almost always due to anticoagulation which is partially out of control. Transfusions were required in 2 patients and bleeding occurred on the third and fifth day, instigated by removal of a Hemovac drain system. In addition, in these patients who bled there was prolonged wound drainage and delayed healing secondary to the hematoma.

It is not clear whether long-term or short-term anticoagulation is essential for the beneficial effects against the tumor. Some believe that short-term anticoagulants (7 days or less) probably only influences blood-borne cancer cells, while long-term therapy may be effective by paralysis of the cancer cell membrane in situ (26). Other possible mechanisms include that vitamin K dependent proteins (other than coagulation factors II, VII, IX, X) requiring gamma carboxyl glutamic acid may be involved in tumor cell interactions with endothelial cells, with normal tissue and/or with other tumor cells.

Other studies have suggested a beneficial effect of anti-coagulation with heparin or coumadin in a variety of different human tumors, particularly lung tumors, and in a variety of unresponsive carcinomas, sarcomas and leukemias (26-29). However, additional studies (30-31) suggest that the use of heparin and chemotherapy have no beneficial effect(s) on the treatment of inoperable lung cancers. In fact, hemorrhage and severe infections were frequent toxic manifestations associated with heparin therapy.

It must be clear to all who have read this article to the end that the study of the role of coagulation and anticoagulants in tumor growth and metastasis is just beginning.

REFERENCES

1. O'Meara, R.A.Q.: Coagulative properties of cancer. Irish J. Med. Sci. 394:474, 1958.

2. O'Meara, R.A.Q. and Jackson, R.D.: Cytological observations on carcinoma. Irish J. Med. Sci. 391:327, 1958.

3. O'Meara, R.A.Q. and Thornes, R.D.: Some properties of cancer coagulative factor. Irish J. Med. Sci. 423:106, 1961.

4. Quigley, H.J.: Peripheral leukocyte thromboplastin in promyelocytic leukemia. Fed. Proc. 26:648 (abstr), 1967.

5. Gralnick, H.R. and Abrell, E.: Studies of the procoagulant and fibrinolytic activity of promyelocytes in acute promyelocytic leukaemia. Brit. J. Haematol. 24:89, 1973.

6. Sakuragawa, N., Takahashi, K., Hoshiyama, M., Jimbo, C., Matsuoka, M. and Onishi, Y.: Pathology cells as procoagulant substance of disseminated intravascular coagulation syndrome in acute promyelocytic leukemia. Thromb. Res. 8:263, 1976.

7. Garg, S. and Niemetz, J.: Tissue factor activity of normal and leukemic cells. Blood 42:729, 1973.

8. Bagnoud, F.: Coagulopathies et carcinomes riche en muco-polysaccharides. Thromb. Diath. Haemorrhag. 15:143, 1966.

9. Pineo, G.F., Regoeczi, E., Hatton, M.W.C. and Brain, M.C.: The activation of coagulation by extracts of mucus; a possible pathway of intravascular coagulation accompanying adenocarcinomas. J. Lab. Clin. Med. 82:255, 1973.

10. Sakuragawa, N., Takahashi, K., Hoshiyama, M., Jimbo, C., Ashizawa, K., Matsuoka, M. and Ohnishi, Y.: The extract from the tissue of gastric cancer as procoagulant in disseminated intravascular coagulation syndrome. Thromb. Res. 10:457, 1977.

11. Gordon, S.G., Franks, J.J. and Lewis, B.: Cancer procoagulant A: A factor X activating procoagulant from malignant tissue. Thromb. Res. 6:127, 1975.

12. Semeraro, N.: Pathways of blood clotting initiation by cancer cells. VIIth Int. Cong. Thromb. Haem., p. 352, 1979.

13. Mohammad, S.F., Moffler, M. and Mason, R.G.: Isolation of a specific procoagulant activity in human lung carcinoma cell lines. VIIth Int. Cong. Thromb. Haem., p. 339, 1979.

14. Laki, K., Csako, G., Yancey, S.T. and Wilson, E.F.: A possible role of transglutaminase in tumor growth and metastases. In, Search and Discovery, Academic Press, Inc., New York, p. 303, 1977.

15. Laki, K., Tyler, H.M. and Yancey, S.T.: Clot forming and clot stabilizing enzymes from the mouse tumor YPC-1. Biochem. Biophys. Res. Comm. 24:776, 1966.

16. Laki, K.: Fakto XIII und metastasierung. In Onkohamostaseologie, H. Gastpar (ed.), F. K. Schattauer Verlag, Stuttgart, Vol. 20, p. 61, 1975.

17. Gralnick, H.R., Bagley, J. and Abrell, E.: Heparin treatment for the hemorrhagic diathesis of acute promyelocytic leukemia. Am. J. Med. 52:167, 1972.

18. Dreyfus, B., Varet, B., Heilmann-Gouault, M., Sultan, C., Reyes, F., Gluckman, E., Basch, A. and Beaujean, F.: Traitment dans 17 observations de leucemies aiques promyelocytaires de la coagulation intravasculaire disseminee. Nouv. Rev. Fr. Hematol. 13:755, 1973.

19. Matsuoka, M. and Watanabe, T.: Studies on the 30 cases of acute promyelocytic leukemia. Jpn. J. Clin. Hematol. 15:1, 1974.

20. Gralnick, H.R. and Sultan, C.: Acute promyelocytic leukemia: Haemorrhagic manifestation and morphologic criteria. Brit. J. Haematol. 29:333, 1975.

21. Gouault-Heilmann, M., Chardon, E., Sultan, C. and Josso, F.: The procoagulant factor of leukaemic promyelocytes: Demonstration of immunologic cross reactivity with human brain tissue factor. Brit. J. Haematol. 30:151, 1975.

22. Drapkin, R.L., Gee, T.S., Dowling, M.D., Arlin, Z., McKenzie, S., Kempin, S. and Clarkson, B.: Prophylactic heparin therapy in acute promyelocytic leukemia. Cancer 41:2484, 1978.

23. Chang, J.C. and Hall, T.C.: In vitro effect of sodium warfarin on DNA and RNA synthesis of mouse L1210 leukemic cells and Walker tumor cells. Oncology 28:232, 1973.

24. Millar, R.C. and Ketcham, A.S.: The effect of heparin and warfarin on primary and metastatic tumors. J. Med. 5:23, 1974.

25. Hoover, H.C., Jr., Ketcham, A.S., Millar, R.C. and Gralnick, H.R.: Osteosarcoma. Improved survival with anticoagulation and amputation. Cancer 41: 2475, 1978.

26. Thornes, R.D.: Oral anticoagulant therapy of human cancer. J. Med. 5:83, 1974.

27. Brown, J.M.: A study of the mechanism by which anticoagulation with warfarin inhibits blood-borne metastases. Cancer Res. 33:1217, 1973.

28. Elias, E.G., Shukia, S.K. and Mink, I.B.: Heparin and chemotherapy in the management of inoperable lung carcinoma. Cancer 36:129, 1975.

29. Hoover, H.C., Jr. and Ketcham, A.S.: Decreasing experimental metastasis formation with anticoagulation and chemotherapy. Surgical Forum 26:173, 1975.

30. Rohwedder, J.J. and Sagastume, E.: Heparin and polychemotherapy for treatment of lung cancer. Cancer Treat. Rep. 61:1399, 1977.

31. Edlis, H.E., Goudsmit, A., Brindley, C. and Niemetz, J.: Trial of heparin and cyclophosphamide (NSC-26271) in the treatment of lung cancer. Cancer Treat. Rep. 60:575, 1976.

Malignancy and the Hemostatic System,
edited by M. B. Donati et al.
Raven Press, New York © 1981.

Pathways of Blood Clotting Initiation by Cancer Cells

N. Semeraro* and M. B. Donati

Istituto di Ricerche Farmacologiche "Mario Negri"
Via Eritrea, 62–20157 Milan, Italy

INTRODUCTION

The involvement of the coagulation system in malignancy has
been strongly suggested by a number of clinical and laboratory
observations. First, malignant disease is associated with a high
incidence of vascular thrombosis or disseminated intravascular
coagulation (DIC) as already recognized by Trousseau (69) more
than a century ago and repeatedly demonstrated by many other clinical studies (1,4,17,33,34,37,66). These coagulation disorders
are most commonly observed in carcinomas (especially mucin-producing adenocarcinoma) of different organs such as the pancreas and
prostate (where the incidence may approach 50%), lung, colon,
stomach, ovary and in acute leukemia (particularly acute promyelocytic leukemia), but they may be seen in any type of cancer.

Other studies have shown that patients with cancer are at "high
risk" for thrombosis or DIC when exposed to various stimuli affecting the hemostatic system. For example, the incidence of
deep venous thrombosis in patients undergoing surgery for cancer
was about 40% (1,55), as compared to 10% in patients without
cancer who underwent comparable surgical procedures (55). Moreover in a group of cancer patients with sepsis the incidence of
DIC was 62% (50).

A number of hemostatic abnormalities, including shortening of
whole blood clotting time in silicone, shortened partial thromboplastin time and prothrombin time, elevated levels of one or more
clotting factors, increased amounts of fibrinogen/fibrin degradation products, presence of circulating fibrin monomers or fibrino-
peptide A, and reduced antithrombin III, have been reported in
malignant disease without clinically evident coagulation disorders
(1,4,37). The most consistent defect was increased platelet and/
or fibrinogen turnover (decreased survival), which was also observed in patients with normal routine coagulation parameters.

----

*Permanent address: Department of Microbiology, Medical School,
University of Bari, Bari, Italy.

Interestingly, these changes were related not only to the presence of active malignant disease but also to the specific type
and extent of disease (35,66). All these findings strongly
suggest that many patients with cancer have low grade intravascular coagulation.

Studies in laboratory animals bearing different types of experimental tumors have also documented the activation of blood clotting mechanisms (8,26,57). In addition, using histochemical,
immunological or radioisotopic techniques, several investigators
have found fibrin deposits in and around the tumor in both human
and experimental malignancies (27,42,47,52,53). It has been
suggested that fibrin might be a suitable stroma for tumor cell
invasion into normal tissues (44,45), though other workers have
postulated that fibrin deposition in tumors might instead be part
of a defence reaction against cell invasiveness (51,52).

In view of the clear involvement of the clotting system in
malignancy, the mechanism(s) of activation of blood coagulation
leading to local or generalized fibrin deposition has been the
topic of extensive investigation during the past three decades.
Its precise understanding could be of great importance not only
for the development of adequate measures for prevention and
treatment of thromboembolic and/or hemorrhagic complications of
malignancy, but also for clarifying the postulated role of fibrin
in tumor growth and metastasis formation.

HOST'S CONTRIBUTION TO FIBRIN FORMATION

There are numerous potential mechanisms by which blood coagulation may be triggered in malignancy. Blood platelets may be
activated by contact with cells from human or experimental tumors
and transformed cells and subsequently aggregate and release their
constituents in vitro and in vivo (13-15, 49, 72). Such platelet
'activation' might lead to unmasking or enhancement of the various
platelet coagulant activities (65,71) and thus contribute to blood
clotting initiation. Mononuclear phagocytes (monocyte/macrophage
cells) could play a similar role since they produce a procoagulant
activity (tissue factor) in response to various stimuli (41).
These cells are an integral part of the lymphoreticular infiltrate
of experimental and human tumors (11,16,73). In addition macrophages isolated from certain tumors are "activated" (36,61).

It is known that most tumors undergo neovascularization; the
potentially abnormal endothelial lining of the neoformed vessels
might be responsible for activation of the contact system, thus
triggering blood clotting through the intrinsic pathway (1). The
destruction of normal tissues during the natural course of tumor
development and subsequent liberation of tissue thromboplastin is
another possible trigger of blood coagulation via the extrinsic
pathway (1). In pancreatic carcinoma the release of systemic
trypsin, which has thrombin-like activity and activates several
coagulation factors, is thought to play a major role (1).

Although these relatively poorly defined mechanisms may be of importance at least in some particular types of cancer, there is clinical and experimental evidence that the most probable cause of the initiation of blood coagulation in malignancy is the production of clot-promoting substances by the cancer cells themselves. This report deals further with current concepts on procoagulant activities of cancer cells and on their mechanisms of action.

CANCER CELL PROCOAGULANT ACTIVITIES

It has long been known that procoagulant activity is present in malignant human tissues and in experimental tumors. About 20 years ago O'Meara (43) first demonstrated that human cancer tissues, particularly carcinomas derived from different organs, consistently caused clotting (not followed by lysis) in normal diluted plasma in the presence of calcium ions; in contrast, normal tissue from the same organs only occasionally induced clotting which was followed by lysis. This increased "coagulative action" associated with diminished fibrinolysis was thought to be responsible for the fibrin deposition seen in human cancers.

Subsequent studies by O'Meara and his associates (2,45,46,48) and by other investigators (15,62,67) have essentially confirmed that human cancers (mostly tissue extracts) do, to various extents, shorten the clotting time of recalcified autologous platelet-poor plasma and are therefore said to possess procoagulant activity. O'Meara et al. (3,46) further investigated the physicochemical properties of this 'cancer coagulative factor' and reported that it was acid, diffusible, and heat-labile. They ultimately concluded that long-chain fatty acids associated with proteins, such as albumin, were responsible for the procoagulant activity.

A similar procoagulant effect was found by several authors in many experimental tumors (tissue homogenates, tissue extracts, single cell suspensions prepared from the tumoral mass or from ascitic fluid or isolated in culture) and this property is reported to vary widely between different experimental tumors or between different forms of the same tumor (15,25,28-31,54).

Although in most studies mentioned above the exact nature and mechanism of action of tumor procoagulant activity was not conclusively established, it was rather non specifically called 'thromboplastic' because, as stated by Boggust et al. (3), "it induces coagulation in recalcified citrated human plasma and is without direct action on fibrinogen alone or on citrated plasma before recalcification". Since a similar procoagulant activity is obtained during extraction of several normal tissues, it was first unclear why in cancer patients or in tumor bearing animals it should induce fibrin formation and deposition. Emphasis was placed mainly on the fact that thromboplastic activity is produced in greater amounts by malignant than normal tissues and that it can easily diffuse in its environment in contrast to normal tissue thromboplastin which diffuses very little unless the tissue is

damaged (28,43,45). Benign tumor extracts were virtually inert
(45). However, there is disagreement about quantitative differences between coagulant activities in malignant and normal tissues
or in malignant and benign tumors. Svanberg (67) reported that
thromboplastic activity is present in similar amounts in benign
and malignant human ovarian tumors although significantly higher
than that of normal ovaries. Holyoke et al. (29) have shown that
cultured T-241 Lewis Sarcoma cells of mouse origin release thromboplastic activity, as measured by recalcification time of mouse
plasma, into their culture medium. However, cultured mouse embryo epithelial or muscle fibroblasts, with no demonstrable
tumorigenic potential, released even more thromboplastic activity
(per mg of total cell protein). In vitro trauma increased the
release of thromboplastic activity from normal and tumor tissues.
In another study with the same tumor Frank and Holyoke (12) used
small millipore collection chambers in vivo to demonstrate that
tissue fluid samples collected from the tumor periphery had more
thromboplastic activity than samples from normal subcutaneous
tissues. It was suggested that this increased clotting activity
might be simply due to mutual destruction of normal and malignant
tissues. Finally Gordon et al. (19) found there were no consistent quantitative differences between normal and malignant human
tissues.

More recent investigations have centered on the question of
qualitative differences between procoagulants from normal and
malignant tissues or from different malignancies with respect to
the mechanism(s) triggering blood clotting.

FACTOR X ACTIVATING ACTIVITY

Some years ago Pineo et al. (55,56) reported that partially
purified mucin from secretions of non-purulent chronic bronchitis,
ovarian cyst fluid and saliva, and extracts of mucin-producing
adenocarcinomas initiated blood coagulation by direct factor VII-
independent activation of coagulation factor X and suggested that
this procoagulant might play a role in the coagulation disorders
of patients with mucus-producing adenocarcinomas. Subsequently
Gordon et al. (18) described a similar activity in extracts from
human malignant tissues and from an experimental tumor (rabbit V_2
carcinoma). This activity appeared to be releated to the presence
in the extracts of a serine protease, called cancer procoagulant
A (CPA), which was inhibited by diisopropyl fluorophosphate (DFP).
Further studies by these investigators, comparing procoagulant
activities in extracts of matched normal and malignant human
tissue samples from the large intestine, breast, lung and kidney,
showed that tumor extracts contained almost exclusively procoagulant activity with the two enzymatic characteristics of CPA
(inhibition by DFP and lack of dependence on F VII) whereas extracts of normal tissues contained typical thromboplastin (F VII-
dependent, insensitive to DFP) (19). All these studies were
performed using tissue extracts, so it was not clear whether pro-

coagulant activity was actually derived from malignant cells.

In order to avoid any interference from connective tissue, muscle, vascular cells or other common contaminants of tumoral masses, we have studied the procoagulant activity of cells from some experimental tumors isolated in culture or as single-cell suspensions from ascitic fluid (5,6). Cells from Lewis Lung carcinoma (3LL), primary and lung metastases, Ehrlich Carcinoma ascites (Eh.ca.) and JW sarcoma ascites (JWS) markedly shortened the recalcification time of normal, factor VIII and factor VII-deficient but not of factor X-deficient human plasma (Table I). The same cells generated thrombin when mixed with a source of prothrombin and factor X, absorbed bovine serum (as a source of factor V), phospholipid and calcium chloride; thrombin formation in this assay was not influenced by the presence of factor VII (6). These findings strongly suggest that cancer cells directly activate coagulation factor X.

More direct evidence for this assumption was obtained in experiments in which cells generated factor Xa, as measured by a specific chromogenic substrate (S-2222), when incubated at 37°C with a source of factor X (BaSO$_4$ eluate from normal or factor VII-deficient serum) and calcium chloride (Table II). The amount of factor Xa formed was independent of factor VII concentration (Table II, Fig. 1) and, at a given cell number, was proportional to the incubation time of the cells-serum eluate-CaCl$_2$ mixture (Fig. 1). Fig. 2 shows the dependence of factor Xa generation upon cell number. Whatever the method used, procoagulant activity was present in the supernatant of active cells (Tables I and II).

Control experiments showed that our assay readily discriminated between direct and factor VII-mediated activation of factor X. Indeed, when cells with thromboplastin-like activity, namely mouse embryo fibroblasts (FET), were tested, the rate of S-2222 cleavage

TABLE I. Effect of cells on plasma recalcification time

Cells (8x10^6/ml)	Plasma recalcification time (sec.)			
	Normal	F VIII-def	F VII —def	F X-def
3LL (Primary)	48	59	50	215
3LL (Supernatant)	64	69	65	258
3LL (Metastasis)	45	51	45	205
Eh.ca.	45	45	48	260
Eh.ca.Supernatant	59	64	62	298
JWS	85	255	87	368
S 180	113	404	129	345
L 929	120	350	140	390
FET	60	55	112	223
Buffer	122-139	488-605	128-139	315-450

TABLE II. F X activation by cells as evaluated by an amidolytic
                                assay (5)

Cells (8x10^6/ml)	S-2222 Cleavage (ΔA 405 nm/5 min)	
	Normal eluate	F VII def Eluate
3LL	.085	.080
Eh.ca.	.100	.092
Eh.ca.Supernatant	.036	.034
S 180	.006	.004
FET	.112	.020
L 929	.000	

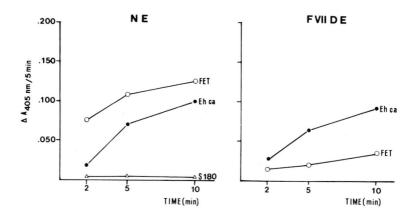

FIG. 1. Dependence of factor Xa formation on the incubation time
         of cells-serum eluate-CaCl$_2$ mixture.

was markedly lower with factor VII-deficient than with normal
serum eluate (Table II, Fig. 1). A similar dependence on factor VII
for FET was shown in the clotting assays (Table I). Cells from
S 180 and control cell line NCTC-1-L929 (L929) were completely
inactive in all test systems employed. These findings provide
evidence on pure cell populations that factor X activating activity may be an intrinsic property of cancer cells and that it may,
at least in part, be released in the surrounding medium.

   That such an activity actually derives from malignant cells was
also demonstrated by Gordon and Lewis (20). These investigators
showed that serum-free medium from cultured malignant cells (V$_2$
carcinoma and parietal yolk sac carcinoma) contained procoagulant
activity that was completely inhibited by DFP and thus met the
basic criteria of CPA. In addition they compared procoagulants

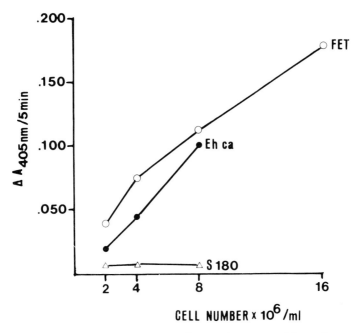

FIG. 2. Dependence of factor Xa formation on cell number.

in serum-free medium from matched normal and SV 40-transformed
hamster embryo fibroblasts and found that procoagulant activity
present in the latter had the enzymatic properties of CPA (DFP-
sensitive serine protease activating factor X in the absence of
factor VII) whereas the normal cells contained procoagulant activity similar to tissue thromboplastin.

Taken altogether, these studies demonstrate that some cancer
cells and transformed cells produce a principle, most probably a
serine protease, capable of directly activating coagulation factor
X; they strongly suggest the existence of an alternative "cellular"
pathway in blood clotting initiation, distinct from both the
intrinsic and extrinsic mechanisms. The same cells contain little,
if any, thromboplastin-like activity which, in contrast, is the
only procoagulant found in normal tissues. There thus seems to be
an apparent loss of tissue thromboplastin activity in malignant
tissues and transformed cells with a concurrent replacement by
CPA activity (19). One might conclude that factor X activating
activity or CPA is a marker of malignancy and that there is a
unique pathway of blood clotting initiation in malignancy (direct
activation of factor X).

However, available evidence indicates that the nature of procoagulant activity may be different in various tumors. It is
worth mentioning that a weak coagulant activity directly activating factor X has been described in human and animal (rabbit, rat,
guinea-pig) platelets (64,65,68).

TISSUE FACTOR ACTIVITY

It is well established that a typical tissue factor activating coagulation factor X through factor VII (extrinsic pathway) may occur in some malignant cells. In man the paradigmatic example is the leukemic cell (21,22,23,63). The production of tissue factor by circulating promyeloblasts in acute promyelocytic leukemia has been regarded as the archetypal contribution of malignant cells to hemostasis and thrombosis (24). Isolated leukemic promyelocytes have potent clot-promoting activity, found mainly in the granular fraction (23). The thromboplastin-like nature of this activity was clearly established not only by the fact that it is demonstrable only in the presence of factor VII and is heat-labile (two properties shared by normal tissue extract activity) but also that it is antigenically related to brain tissue factor (21,23). The presence of tissue factor in leukemic promyelocytes is consistent with the high incidence of the DIC syndrome in acute promyelocytic leukemia. It is worth mentioning that freshly isolated normal leucocytes have minimal, if any, procoagulant activity. It is only after appropriate <u>in vitro</u> or <u>in vivo</u> stimulation that they generate a potent procoagulant which has been identified as tissue factor (41). The mononuclear phagocyte (monocyte/macrophage) is the cell primarily involved (10,59). Well known stimulating agents include bacterial endotoxin, phytohemagglutinin, platelets and platelet membranes, antigen-antibody complexes, sensitized lymphocytes, adherence to various surfaces including vascular surfaces, renal dialysis membranes, C5 chemotactic fragment and C3b (38, 41, 58, 60, 70). There is evidence that leucocytes' procoagulant activity may play an important role in DIC induced by endotoxin, in experimental venous thrombosis and in fibrin deposition occurring in some immunological diseases (9,32,39). A clot-promoting activity with the characteristics of tissue factor (factor VII dependence) was also found in cells from an experimental leukemia, rat BNML leukemia (40, Mussoni et al., unpublished). These findings are of interest in view of the fact that signs of intravascular activation of the clotting system were observed in BNML leukemia bearing rats (7). Finally, typical tissue factor was present in some solid tumors such as Walker 256 carcinosarcoma (Semeraro et al., unpublished) and others (30).

In conclusion there are at least two pathways of blood clotting initiation by cancer cells (direct activation of factor X and extrinsic pathway) both requiring calcium ions as schematically represented in Fig. 3. The possible pathophysiological implications of cancer procoagulant activities are not yet well defined. They may conceivably contribute to intravascular activation of blood coagulation in patients with malignant diseases or in tumor-bearing animals. They may also play a role in tumor growth and dissemination by promoting fibrin deposition. That procoagulant activities may indeed influence the localization of fibrin on tumor tissue is supported by studies on the uptake of intra-

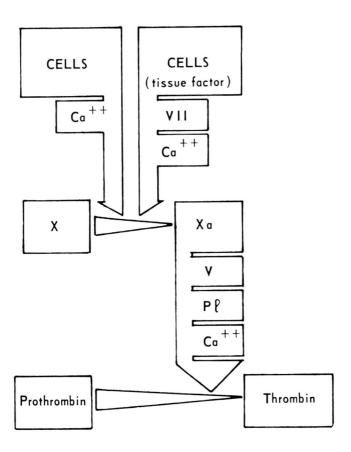

FIG. 3. Pathways of blood clotting initiation by cancer cells.

vascular injected labelled fibrinogen in two mouse tumors (53).
Tumor tissue from a mouse mammary carcinoma with high thromboplastic activity showed greater uptake of labelled fibrinogen
than that of a mouse sarcoma with low coagulant activity.

Even more difficult, with the knowledge available, is how to
establish the relative importance of the two pathways described in
determining these phenomena. As mentioned above we found the same
type of procoagulant in two metastasizing tumors (Lewis lung carcinoma and JW sarcoma) and Ehrlich carcinoma but no procoagulant
activity in S 180 cells (5,6). These data therefore do not suggest any clear relation between this activity and cell invasiveness. Gordon and Lewis (20) found no apparent correlation between
specific procoagulant activity (CPA) and tumorigenicity of transformed fibroblasts.

Clearly more controlled in vitro studies for characterization
and quantitation of coagulant activities and in vivo studies using
cells with well defined procoagulant activity are required to shed

fresh light in this interesting field.

ACKNOWLEDGEMENTS

The authors' work mentioned in this review has been partially supported by Grant NIH-PHRB-1RO1 CA L2764-01, National Cancer Institute, NIH, Bethesda, Maryland, USA and by Contract 78.02.798.96, Italian National Research Council, Rome, Italy.
    Judith Baggott, Vincenzo de Ceglie, Paola Bonifacino and Anna Mancini helped prepare the manuscript.

REFERENCES

1. Bick, R.L. (1978): Alterations of hemostasis associated with malignancy: Etiology, pathophysiology, diagnosis and management. Semin. Thromb. Hemostas., 5:1-26.

2. Boggust, W.A., O'Brien, D.J., O'Meara, R.A.Q., and Thornes, R.D. (1963): The coagulative factors of normal human and human cancer tissue. Ir. J. Med. Sci., 477: 131-144.

3. Boggust, W.A., O'Meara, R.A.Q., and Fullerton, W.W. (1968): Diffusible thrombloplastins of human cancer and chorion tissue. Eur. J. Cancer, 3:467-473.

4. Brugarolas, A., Mink, I.B., Elias, E.G., and Mittelman, A. (1973): Correlation of hyperfibrinogenemia with major thromboembolism in patients with cancer. Surg.Gynecol. Obstet., 136: 75-77.

5. Colucci, M., Curatolo, L., Donati, M.B., and Semeraro, N. (1979): Direct activation of factor X by some cancer cells: Evaluation by an amidolytic assay. Thromb. Haemost.,42:167.

6. Curatolo, L., Colucci, M., Cambini, A.L., Poggi,A., Morasca, L., Donati, M.B., and Semeraro, N. (1979): Evidence that cells from experimental tumours can activate coagulation factor X. Br. J. Cancer, 40: 228-233.

7. Donati, M.B., Mussoni, L., Kornblihtt, L., and Poggi, A. (1977): Changes in the hemostatic system of rats bearing L5222 or BNML experimental leukemias. Leukemia Res., 1:177-180.

8. Donati, M.B., Poggi, A., Mussoni, L., de Gaetano, G., and
   Garattini, S. (1977):Hemostasis and experimental cancer
   dissemination. In: <u>Cancer Invasion and Metastasis:Biologic
   Mechanisms and Therapy</u>, edited by S.B. Day, W.P.L. Myers,
   P. Stansly, S. Garattini, and M.G. Lewis, pp. 151-160.
   Raven Press, New York.

9. Edwards, R.L., and Rickles, F.R. (1978): Delayed hypersensitivity in man: Effects of systemic anticoagulation.
   <u>Science</u>, 200:541-543.

10. Edwards, R.L., Rickles, F.R., and Bobrove, A.M. (1979):
    Mononuclear cell tissue factor: Cell of origin and
    requirements for activation. <u>Blood</u>, 54:359-370.

11. Evans, R. (1972): Macrophages in syngeneic animal tumours.
    <u>Transplantation</u>, 14:468-473.

12. Frank, A.L., and Holyoke, E.D. (1968): Tumor fluid thrombo-
    plastin activity. <u>Int. J. Cancer</u>, 3:677-682.

13. Gasic, G.J., Boettiger, D., Catalfamo, J.L., Gasic, T.B.,
    and Stewart, G.J. (1978): Aggregation of platelets and
    cell membrane vesiculation by rat cells, transformed "in
    vitro" by Rous sarcoma virus. <u>Cancer Res.</u>, 38:2950-2955.

14. Gasic, G.J., Boettiger, D., Catalfamo, J.L., Gasic, T.B.,
    and Stewart, G.J. (1978): Platelet interactions in
    malignancy and cell transformation: Functional and
    biochemical studies. In: <u>Platelets: A Multidisciplinary
    Approach</u>, edited by G. de Gaetano, and S. Garattini,
    pp.447-456. Raven Press, New York.

15. Gasic, G.J., Koch, P.A.G., Hsu, B., Gasic, T.B., and
    Niewiarowski, S. (1976): Thrombogenic activity of mouse
    and human tumors: Effects on platelets, coagulation and
    fibrinolysis, and possible significance for metastases.
    <u>Z. Krebsforsch.</u>, 86:263-277.

16. Gauci, C.L., and Alexander, P. (1975): The macrophage
    content of some human tumours.<u>Cancer Lett.</u>, 1:29-32.

17. Goodnight, S.H.Jr. (1974): Bleeding and intravascular clotting in malignancy: A review. Ann. N.Y. Acad. Sci., 230:271-288.

18. Gordon, S.G., Franks, J.J., and Lewis, B. (1975): Cancer procoagulant A: A factor X activating procoagulant from malignant tissue. Thromb. Res., 6:127-137.

19. Gordon, S.G., Franks, J.J., and Lewis, B.J. (1979): Comparison of procoagulant activities in extracts of normal and malignant human tissue. J. Natl. Cancer Inst., 62:773-776.

20. Gordon, S.G., and Lewis,B.J.(1978):Comparison of procoagulant activity in tissue culture medium from normal and transformed fibroblasts. Cancer Res., 38:2467-2472.

21. Gouault-Heilmann, M., Chardon, E., Sultan, C., and Josso, F. (1975): The procoagulant factor of leukaemic promyelocytes: Demonstration of immunologic cross reactivity with human brain tissue factor. Br. J. Haematol., 30:151-158.

22. Gralnick, H.R. (1979): Cancer cell procoagulant activity. Thromb. Haemostas., 42:352.

23. Gralnick,H.R., and Abrell, E. (1973): Studies on the procoagulant and fibrinolytic activity of promyelocytes in acute promyelocytic leukaemia. Br. J. Haematol.,24:89-99.

24. Gralnick, H.R., and Tan, H.K. (1974): Acute promyelocytic leukemia. A model for understanding the role of the malignant cell in hemostasis. Hum. Pathol., 5:661-673.

25. Hilgard, P., and Hiemeyer, V. (1970): Fibrinolysis,thromboplastin activity and localization of radioiodinated fibrinogen in experimental tumors. Eur. J. Cancer,6;157-158.

26. Hilgard, P., Hohage, R., Schmitt, W., and Kühle, W. (1973): Microangiopathic haemolytic anaemia associated with hypercalcaemia in an experimental rat tumour.Br. J. Haematol., 24:245-254.

27. Hiramoto, R., Bernecky, J., Jurandowski, J., Pressman, D. (1960): Fibrin in human tumors. Cancer Res.,20:592-593.

28. Holyoke, E.D., and Ichihashi, H. (1966): The C3H/St/Ha mammary tumor. I. Thromboplastin content. J. Natl. Cancer Inst., 36:1049-1055.

29. Holyoke, E.D., Frank, A.L., and Weiss, L. (1972): Tumor thromboplastin activity "in vitro". Int. J. Cancer, 9:258-263.

30. Khato, J., Suzuki, M., and Sato, H. (1974): Quantitative study on thromboplastin in various strains of Yoshida ascites hepatoma cells of rat. Gan., 65:289-294.

31. Lawrence, E.A., Bowman, D.E., Moore, D.B., and Bernstein, G.I. (1954): A thromboplastic property of neoplasms. Surg. Forum, 3:694-698.

32. Lerner, R.G., Goldstein, R., and Nelson, J.C. (1977): Production of thromboplastin (tissue factor) and thrombi by polymorphonuclear neutrophilic leukocytes adhering to vein walls. Thromb. Res., 11:11-22.

33. Lieberman, J.S., Borrero, J., Urdaneta, E., and Wright, I.S. (1961): Thrombophlebitis and cancer. J.A.M.A., 177:542-545.

34. Lisiewicz, J. (1978): Mechanisms of hemorrhage in leukemias. Semin. Thromb. Hemostas.,4:241-267.

35. Lyman, G.H., Bettigole, R.E., Robson, E., Ambrus, J.L., and Urban, H. (1978): Fibrinogen kinetics in patients with neoplastic disease. Cancer, 41:1113-1122.

36. Mantovani, A. (1978): Effects on "in vitro" tumor growth of murine macrophages isolated from sarcoma lines differing in immunogenicity and metastasizing capacity. Int. J. Cancer,22:741-746.

37. Miller, S.P., Sanchez-Avalos, J., Stafanski, T., and Zuckerman, L. (1967): Coagulation disorders in cancer. I. Clinical and laboratory studies. Cancer, 20:1452-1465.

38. Muhlfelder, T.W., Niemetz, J., Kreutzer, D., Beebe, D., Ward, P.A., and Rosenfeld, S.I. (1979): C5 chemotactic fragment induces leucocyte production of tissue factor activity. A link between complement and coagulation. J. Clin. Invest., 63:147-150.

39. Müller-Berghaus, G. (1978): The role of platelets,leukocytes, and complement in the activation of intravascular coagulation by endotoxin. In: Platelets:A Multidisciplinary Approach, edited by G. de Gaetano, and S. Garattini, pp.303-320. Raven Press, New York.

40. Mussoni, L., Bertoni, M.P., Curatolo, L., Poggi, A., and Donati, M.B. (1977): "In vitro" interactions of L5222 and BNML leukemia cells with fibrin. A preliminary report. Leukemia Res., 1:181-183.

41. Niemetz, J., Mühlfelder, T., Chierego, M.E., and Troy, B. (1977): Procoagulant activity of leukocytes. Ann. N.Y. Acad. Sci., 283:208-217.

42. Ogura, T., Tsubura, E., and Yamamura, Y. (1970):Localization of radioiodinated fibrinogen in invaded and metastasized tumor tissue of Walker carcinosarcoma. Gan., 61:443-449.

43. O'Meara, R.A.Q. (1958): Coagulative properties of cancers. Ir. J. Med. Sci., no.394:474-479.

44. O'Meara, R.A.Q. (1968): Fibrin formation and tumour growth. Thromb. Diath. Haemorrh., Suppl. 28:137-146.

45. O'Meara, R.A.Q. (1969): Thrombloplastic materials from human tumours and chorion. In: Ciba Foundation Symposium on Homeostatic Regulators, edited by G.E.W. Wolstenholme, and J. Knight, pp. 85-97. J. & A. Churchill Ltd., London.

46. O'Meara, R.A.Q. (1970): Cancer research at Saint Luke's Hospital. Ir. J. Med. Sci., 3:59-65.

47. O'Meara, R.A.Q., and Jackson, R.D. (1958): Cytological observations on carcinoma. Ir. J. Med. Sci.,no.391:327-328.

48. O'Meara, R.A.Q., and Thornes, R.D. (1961): Some properties of the cancer coagulative factor. Ir. J. Med. Sci., no. 423:106-112.

49. Pearlstein, E., Cooper, L.B., and Karpatkin, S. (1980): Extraction and characterization of a platelet aggregating material (PAM) from SV40-transformed mouse 3T3 fibroblasts. J. Lab. Clin. Med., in press.

50. Peck, S.D., and Reiquam, C.W. (1973) : Disseminated intravascular coagulation in cancer patients: Supportive evidence. Cancer, 31:1114-1119.

51. Peterson, H.I. (1968): Experimental studies on fibrinolysis in growth and spread of tumour. Acta Chir. Scand. Suppl.394.

52. Peterson, H.I. (1977): Fibrinolysis and antifibrinolytic drugs in the growth and spread of tumours. Cancer Treat. Rev., 4:213-217.

53. Peterson, H.I., Appelgren, K.L., and Rosengren, B.H.O. (1969): Fibrinogen metabolism in experimental tumours. Eur. J. Cancer, 5: 535-542.

54. Peterson, H.I., and Zettergren, L. (1970): Thromboplastic and fibrinolytic properties of three transplantable rat tumours. Acta Chir. Scand., 136: 365-368.

55. Pineo, G.F., Brain, M.C., Gallus, A.S., Hirsh, J., Hatton, M.W.C., and Regoeczi, E. (1974): Tumors mucus production, and hypercoagulability. Ann. N.Y. Acad. Sci.,230:262-270.

56. Pineo, G.F., Regoeczi, E., Hatton, M.W.C., and Brain, M.C. (1973): The activation of coagulation by extracts of mucus: A possible pathway of intravascular coagulation accompanying adenocarcinomas. J. Lab. Clin. Med., 82:255-266.

57. Poggi, A., Polentarutti, N., Donati, M.B., de Gaetano, G., and Garattini, S. (1977): Blood coagulation changes in mice bearing Lewis lung carcinoma, a metastasizing tumor. Cancer Res., 37:272-277.

58. Prydz, H., Allison, A.C., and Schorlemmer, H.U. (1977): Further link between complement activation and blood coagulation. Nature, 270:173-174.

59. Rivers, R.P.A., Hathaway, W.E., and Weston, W.L. (1975): The endotoxin-induced coagulant activity of human monocytes. Br. J. Haematol., 30:311-316.

60. Rothberger, H., Zimmerman, T.S., Spiegelberg, H.L., and Vaughan, J.H. (1977): Leukocyte procoagulant activity. Enhancement of production in vitro by IgG and antigen-antibody complexes. J. Clin. Invest., 59:549-557.

61. Russell, S.W., Doe, W.F., and McIntosh, A.T. (1977): Functional characterization of a stable, noncytolytic stage of macrophage activation in tumors. J. Exp. Med., 146:1511-1520.

62. Sakuragawa, N., Takahashi, K., Hoshiyama, M., Jimbo, C., Ashizawa, K., Matsuoka, M., and Ohnishi, Y. (1977): The extract from the tissue of gastric cancer as procoagulant in disseminated intravascular coagulation syndrome. Thromb. Res., 10:457-463.

63. Sakuragawa, N., Takahashi, K., Hoshiyama, M., Jimbo, C., Matsuoka, M., and Onishi, Y. (1976): Pathologic cells as procoagulant substance of disseminated intravascular coagulation syndrome in acute promyelocytic leukemia. Thromb. Res., 8:263-273.

64. Semeraro, N., Colucci, M., and Vermylen, J. (1979): Complement-dependent and complement-independent interactions of bacterial lipopolysaccharides and mucopeptides with rabbit and human platelets. Thromb. Haemost., 41:392-406.

65. Semeraro, N., and Vermylen, J. (1977): Evidence that washed human platelets possess factor-X activator activity. Br. J. Haematol., 36:107-115.

66. Slichter, S.J., and Harker, L.A. (1974): Hemostasis in malignancy. Ann. N.Y. Acad. Sci., 230:252-261.

67. Svanberg, L. (1975): Thromboplastic activity of human ovarian tumours. Thromb. Res., 6:307-313.

68. Tremoli, E., Donati, M.B., and de Gaetano, G. (1977): Washed guinea-pig and rat platelets possess factor-X activator activity. Br. J. Haematol., 37:155-156.

69. Trousseau, A. (1865): Phlegmasia alba dolens. In: Clinique Médicale de l'Hôtel-Dieu de Paris, 3:654-656. Ballière, Paris.

70. van Ginkel, C.J.W., van Aken, W.G., Oh, J.I.H., and Vreeken, J. (1977): Stimulation of monocyte procoagulant activity by adherence to different surfaces. Br. J. Haematol., 37:35-45.

71. Walsh, P.N. (1974): Platelet coagulant activities and haemostasis: A hypothesis. Blood, 43:597-605.

72. Warren, B.A. (1978): Platelet-tumor cell interactions: Morphological studies. In: Platelets: A Multidisciplinary Approach, edited by G. de Gaetano, and S. Garattini, pp.427-446. Raven Press, New York.

73. Wood, G.W., and Gollahon, K.A. (1977): Detection and quantitation of macrophage infiltration into primary human tumors with the use of cell-surface markers. J. Natl. Cancer Inst., 59:1081-1087.

Malignancy and the Hemostatic System,
edited by M. B. Donati et al.
Raven Press, New York © 1981.

Plasminogen Activator Released from Malignant Ovarian Tumours

B. Astedt

Departments of Gynecology and Obstetrics in Malmo and Lund,
University of Lund, S-22185 Lund, Sweden

Malignant tumours possess coagulative properties (5, 8) resulting in deposits of fibrin surrounding tumour formations. These fibrin deposits are a necessary matrix for proliferating neoplastic vessels. Thus, in analogy with the process of tissue repair residual fibrin has to be removed by the fibrinolytic system initiated by plasminogen activators released from the tumour cells (6, 9).

It has been shown that in tissue culture of certain animal cell lines barely any or no detectable amounts of plasminogen activators are released. But if the cells are transformed by oncogenic viruses or carcinogenic substances, they start to produce abundant amounts of plasminogen activators not released by the parent cultures (3, 7). We have shown that the amount of plasminogen activators released in organ culture of normal human ovarian tissue is barely demonstrable. In contrast the amounts released in tissue culture of malignant tumours originating in the same organ are large (9). Furthermore, it has been shown that the tumour plasminogen activator is very similar to urokinase. Both are serine proteases and occur in three molecular forms of about 90,000, 54,000 and 31,000 daltons. They are immunologically identical (1, 2).

In view of the immunologic identity a radioimmunoassay for urokinase was devised with the use of monospecific antiurokinase and applied for detection of the tumour plasminogen activator as a biological marker for neoplasia.

MATERIAL AND METHODS

Urokinase

Urokinase (UK) was purified by affinity chromatography on para-aminobenzamidine, carbodiimide coupled to CH-Sepharose 4B (4) followed by gel filtration on Sephadex G-100 Superfine.

In the preparation of the affinity column, 150 mg p-aminobenzamidine (Sigma, USA) was coupled by water soluble carbodiimide to 7.5 g CH-Sepharose 4B (Pharmacia Fine Chemicals, Uppsala). The gel was equilibrated with 0.1 M sodium phosphate buffer, pH 7.0, and 0.4 M NaCl and packed in a 1.6 x 40 cm column to a height of about 12 cm. The starting material consisted of 100,000 Ploug units of Urokinase Reagent (Leo Pharmaceutical Products, Denmark) dissolved in the same buffer as that used for equilibration of the gel. UK was eluted by changing the buffer to 0.1 M acetate, pH 4.0, and 0.4 M NaCl.

The purified UK-preparation was separated by gel chromatography on Sephadex G-100 Superfine (Pharmacia Fine Chemicals, Uppsala) into two molecular fractions of 31,000 and 54,000 daltons. The 31,000 dalton fraction gave only one visible band when analyzed in sodium dodecyl sulfate polyacrylamide gel electrophoresis. It was used for immunization of rabbits, and after inactivation with diisopropylfluorophosphate (DFP), for radioiodination in the radioimmunoassay.

Urokinase antiserum

Rabbits were immunized according to Holmberg et al. (4). The antiserum was harvested after two months.

Labelled urokinase

^{125}I-urokinase was prepared with the lactoperoxidase method according to Thorell and Johansson (11) with the following modifications: 0.2 mg of the purified urokinase dissolved in 1 ml of 0.075 M Tris · HCl (pH 7.5) was inactivated by incubation with 100 ul of 10^{-2} M DFP in propylene glycol for 3 hours. Non-reacted DFP was removed by gel filtration on a small column of Sephadex G-25 (Pharmacia Fine Chemicals, Uppsala). 0.02 mg of DIP-urokinase was iodinated with 1 mCi ^{125}I (IMS 30, Radiochemical Center, Amersham). The total reaction mixture was 115 ul and the reaction time 60 seconds. The ^{125}I DIP-urokinase was purified on small Sephadex G-25 columns. The yield of the iodination was in the range of 20-40 %.

Radioimmunoassay

Radioimmunoassay of UK was performed with a double antibody system. Each tube contained 0.2 ml antiserum diluted 1:20,000, 0.2 ml ^{125}I DIP-urokinase (approx. 0.3 ng) and 0.1 ml standard UK or sample. The tubes were incubated at 4°C for two days, after which 0.05 ml of 1:250 diluted normal rabbit serum and 0.05 ml of 1:10 diluted goat antiserum to rabbit IgG were added.

After addition of 0.1 ml normal plasma to the standard or samples, the tubes were incubated for another 4-18 hours at 4°C. The radioactivity of the precipitate was counted after centrifugation and decanting of the supernatant. For detection of low concentrations of UK-like plasminogen activators the method was made more sensitive by two days´ preincubation of antiserum and sample before addition of ^{125}I DIP-urokinase.

Urokinase in peripheral blood

Twelve thousand Ploug units of purified urokinase were administered to a healthy volunteer (author) and blood samples were taken before administration and continually for 4 hours for examination in the radioimmunoassay. The fibrinolytic activity of the plasma was estimated also on fibrin plates containing plasminogen.

Blood from human ovarian carcinomas

Blood samples were obtained at laparotomy from vessels draining ovarian tumours for estimation of antiurokinase reacting material with the radioimmunoassay. At the same time samples of peripheral venous blood were taken.

Wash from the uterine cavity

Using a jet wash technique the uterine cavity was washed out with a predetermined volume of physiological saline. Curettage was then performed and the endometrium specimens were examined histologically.

RESULTS

The concentrations in the peripheral blood of urokinase administered intravenously to a healthy volunteer, are given in Table I. The initial concentration of urokinase after the intravenous infusion was 33 ng/ml. After a period of 4 hours it was only 6 ng/ml. The enzyme activity on fibrin plates was hardly detectable.

In the blood of veins draining various tumours the concentration of urokinase reacting material was 10 to 25 ng/ml compared with 4 to 6 ng/ml in peripheral blood (Table II).

In the wash from the uterine cavity in patients with malignant histology, the concentration of antiurokinase reacting material was higher than in unaffected cavities (Table III).

TABLE I Radioimmunologically demonstrated fibrino-
lytical activity in peripheral blood following i.v. injection of urokinase

Time (min)	5	15	30	60	120	240
Concentration (ng/ml)	34	22	15	10	6	6
Fibrinolytic activity (Ploug units)	2.2	2	1	0	0	0

TABLE II Radioimmunoassay of plasminogen activator
in blood from patients with ovarian tumours
(ng/ml)

Ovarian tumour	Peripheral venous blood	Blood from vessels draining the tumour
Serous cystadenocarcinoma	5	12
"	5	12
"	5	16
"	4	24
Endometroid adenocarcinoma	6	16
Non-malignant cystoma (5 cases)	4-5	4-6

TABLE III Plasminogen activator in uterine washings

Histologic diagnosis	Concentration ng/ml
Adenocarcinoma	84
"	21
"	16
"	17
Adenoacanthoma (malignant)	>100
Normal endometrium (5 cases)	5-9

DISCUSSION

The results show that the infused urokinase can be easily detected and determined in the radioimmuno-assay. Also in the blood from veins draining malignant tumours the concentrations were higher than in peripheral blood. The values, 4-6 ng/ml, found in peripheral blood resembled those in such blood from healthy persons and were probably due to the background activity. Thus, the radioimmunoassay is not sensitive enough to detect tumour plasminogen activators when diluted in the whole blood volume of the organism. Furthermore, the tumour plasminogen activators are bound to the various naturally occurring inhibitors, which thereby mask the immunological site of the activator molecule.

The enhanced concentration of plasminogen activators in the uterine wash from patients with endometrial carcinoma is in agreement with those found in tissue cultures. The concentrations in the medium of such cultures are high if the endometrium is cancerous, but low if it is normal(10). Cytologic examination is of limited diagnostic value in endometrial neoplasia. The present results indicate that the radioimmunoassay of antiurokinase reacting material in the uterine wash would be more helpful.

The urokinase molecule with a molecular weight of 54.000 daltons contains a heavy chain of about 30,000 daltons and a light chain of about 20,000 daltons. The active site is situated in the heavy chain (4). Recently we succeeded in raising an antiserum against the light chain of the urokinase molecule. Also between the light chain of the urokinase molecule and the tumour plasminogen activator molecule there is immunologic identity. The naturally occurring inhibitors do not bind to the light chain, which is probably circulating free in the blood in patients with neoplasia. Thus, the antibodies against the light chain will, perhaps, prove more useful for detecting the tumour plasminogen activator.

ACKNOWLEDGEMENT

This work was supported by grant B80-17X-04523-06C from the Swedish Medical Research Council.

REFERENCES

1. Åstedt, B., and Holmberg, L. (1976): Immunological identity of urokinase and ovarian carcinoma plasminogen activator released in tissue culture. Nature 261:595.

2. Åstedt, B., Lundgren, E., Roos, G., and Abu Sinna, G. (1978): Release of various molecular forms of plasminogen activators during culture of human ovarian tumours. Thromb. Res. 13:1031.

3. Christman, J., and Acs, G. (1974): Purification and characterization of a cellular fibrinolytic factor associated with oncogenic transformation: the plasminogen activator from SV-40-transformed hamster cells. Biochim.Biophys.Acta 340:339.

4. Holmberg, L., Bladh, B., and Åstedt, B. (1976): Purification of urokinase by affinity chromatography. Biochim. Biophys. Acta 445:215.

5. O´Meara, R.A.Q., and Thornes, R.D. (1961): Some properties of the cancer coagulative factor. Irish J. Med. Sci. 423:106.

6. Reich, E. (1975): Plasminogen activator: Secretion by neoplastic cells and macrophages. In "Proteases and Biological Control". Cold Spring Harbor Laboratory.

7. Rifkin, D., Loeb, J., Moore, G., and Reich, E. (1974): Properties of plasminogen activators formed by neoplastic human cell cultures. J.Exp.Med. 139:1317.

8. Svanberg, L. (1975): Thromboplastic activity of human ovarian tumours. Thromb. Res. 6:307.

9. Svanberg, L., and Åstedt, B. (1976): Release of fibrinolytic activators from human ovarian tumours in organ culture. Ann. Chir. et Gynaec. 65:405.

10. Svanberg, L., and Åstedt, B. Release of plasminogen activator from normal and neoplastic endometrium. Experientia. In press.

11. Thorell, J.I., and Johansson, B.G. (1971): Enzymatic iodination of polypeptides with ^{125}I to high specific activity. Biochim.Biophys.Acta 251:363.

Malignancy and the Hemostatic System,
edited by M. B. Donati et al.
Raven Press, New York © 1981.

Fibrin and Cancer Cell Growth:
Problems in the Evaluation of Experimental Models

Andreina Poggi, Maria Benedetta Donati, and Silvio Garattini

Istituto di Ricerche Farmacologiche "Mario Negri"
Via Eritrea, 62-20157 Milan, Italy

INTRODUCTION

Over the past 20 years the concept of fibrin playing a role
in cancer cell growth and dissemination has received some experimental support, although indirect, from animal models.   Such
treatments as antiaggregating, anticoagulant or fibrinolytic
agents have been found to reduce metastasis formation in some
animal models (7).   On the other hand, conditions promoting hypercoagulability, such as hyperlipemia, inhibition of fibrinolysis
or injection of procoagulants have been indicated to favor
metastasis growth (38).   However, the fact remains that many of
the results are still controversial and both the suitability of
the models and the benefit of the therapeutic approaches with
drugs active on hemostasis have been questioned (8,35).

The aim of this paper is first to make a critical evaluation
of the experimental models of dissemination used so far to study
the involvement of the hemostatic system.   The second part
discusses the possibility of controlling tumor growth through
pharmacological modulation of the host's hemostatic components.

ANIMAL MODELS OF DISSEMINATION

Choice of Appropriate Models

Well defined conditions as close as possible to the modalities
of development of clinical tumors should be selected in studies
of the role of hemostatic system factors in cancer growth and
dissemination.   Several long-term experiments have been carried
out with allogenic instead of syngeneic tumors, leaving the possibility that uncontrolled immunological factors may have influenced the results.   Moreover, most of the information on cancer
procoagulants have been obtained in artificial models of tumor
growth, such as hematogenous dissemination following intravenous
(i.v.) injection of cancer cells. In these conditions tumor

89

emboli, rather than real metastases, are formed through a process which by-passes the first steps of local tumor invasion, such as development of cell proteolytic and/or migratory properties, detachment from the primary site and penetration through the vascular walls into the circulation. A rapid i.v. injection of Walker 256 Carcinosarcoma cells in allogenic rats has been described as inducing acute coagulopathy, characterized by raised plasma hemoglobin levels, a fall in peripheral platelet count, and a moderate reduction of plasma fibrinogen levels (15). Sequestration of radio-labelled fibrinogen and platelets in the lungs of the same animals was also demonstrated. However, the lack of specificity of this reaction is indicated by the fact that the injection of dead cells or of particulate, inert, material can induce the same coagulopathy (12). This should be due to activation of the coagulation cascade through the contact phase or to the introduction into the circulation of tissue-derived thromboplastic material.

In our studies, we have shown that i.v. injection of cells from Lewis Lung Carcinoma (3LL) in syngeneic mice induced dose-dependent thrombocytopenia (28). Reduction of fibrinogen levels and increase in fibrin(ogen) degradation products, with no changes in erythrocyte counts were found, starting five minutes after the injection of 4×10^5 3LL cells (30). These changes were rapidly reversible (within one hour), and none of them could be observed at a later stage, when metastatic nodules to the lungs had grown (8).

Pretreating the animals with platelet aggregation inhibitors (aspirin, ditazole) or anticoagulants (warfarin, heparin) prevented these acute hemostatic changes (8,24,25). However it is not yet cearly established whether the acute coagulopathy following i.v. injection of cancer cells plays an important role in lodgement and subsequent lung colony growth.

Blood Coagulation Changes During Tumor Growth

The involvement of the hemostatic system during the growth of experimental tumors has been considered only in a few models. Microangiopathic hemolytic anemia, associated with chronic intravascular coagulation, has been shown to occur in rats bearing intramuscularly (i.m.) implanted, non-disseminating Walker 256 carcinosarcoma (17). Mild intravascular coagulation, with microangiopathic hemolytic anemia, thrombocytopenia (mainly due to impaired synthesis) and raised fibrinogen levels with increased fibrinogen turnover were found in association with the development of a spontaneously metastasizing tumor, the 3LL in syngeneic mice (30). These changes were not abolished by chronic treatment with antiaggregating agents or anticoagulants and did not appear to have a clear pathogenetic link to metastasis formation, since they were also observed in animals treated with warfarin, in which metastatic growth was markedly inhibited (29) (Table I). Moreover although they occurred mainly in concomitance with the growth of

Table 1. Occurrence of thrombocytopenia, anemia and hyperfibrinogenemia in different experimental conditions of 3LL
growth.

	i.m.	i.m.+warfarin	i.m.+ amputation	e.v.
Platelet	↓	↓	→	→
Red cell	↓	↓	→	→
Fibrinogen	↑	↑	→	→
Primary	+	+	−	−
Metastases	+	−	+	+

i.m. = spontaneous metastasis after i.m. implantation of tumor
cells.

i.m. + warfarin = chronic warfarin treatment during the whole
period of tumor development after i.m. implantation of
cells.

i.m. + amputation = amputation of primary tumor at a time (day
7-9) when spontaneous metastases have already started to
develop.

e.v. = lung colony formation after e.v. injection of tumor cells.

the metastases, hemostatic changes in 3LL appeared closely related
to the presence of the primary tumor because, as indicated by the
observations summarized in Table 1, no changes were detected when
lung metastases occurred in the absence of the primary as in the
artificial metastasis model or in the spontaneous model after
removal of the primary at adequate times after tumor implantation.
These data suggest that the presence of the primary tumor unique-
ly influences the host's hemostatic system.

As regards microangiopathy signs, possibly circulation of blood
through the complex network of primary tumor vasculature is
enough to lead to hemolytic anemia; on the other hand, some
inflammatory or toxic substance released from the primary could
depress platelet production. It has been suggested that the
primary tumor exerts an inhibitory effect on the growth of
metastatic nodules through a still undefined mediator (37). It
is not known whether a similar mechanism operates towards blood
platelet production.

The experience so far available on the involvement of the
host's hemostatic system in spontaneous metastasis models is too
limited to establish whether differences in the changes observed
depend on the host's reactivity or on specific cancer cell properties.

Different hemostatic changes can be observed in different experimental tumors. Data on the only two murine metastasizing
tumors so far characterized are presented in Table 2: the 3LL and

Table 2. <u>Characteristics and blood coagulation changes of two different spontaneously metastasizing tumors in mice, the 3LL and the JWS (4,5,21,30)</u>

	C57B1/6J	Balb/c
– Syngeneic strain	C57B1/6J	Balb/c
– Original histological type	adenocarcinoma	sarcoma
– Primary and metastatic growth	encapsulated	infiltrative
– Immunogenicity	weak	strong
– Blood platelet	↓	↓
– Red blood cell	↓	→
– Blood fibrinogen	↑	↑
– Survival time of radiolabelled fibrinogen	↓	→
– Fibrin accumulation in the tumor	+	−
– Blood supply to the tumor (%/g)	+	+
– Cell procoagulant activity	++	+
– Cell fibrinolytic activity	+	++

and the JW Sarcoma (JWS, a recently described tumor) grow in different mouse strains and, when injected s.c. or i.m. both can give spontaneous metastases selectively to the lungs. However, 3LL secondary nodules are encapsulated and readily enucleated from the lungs, whereas JWS metastases are infiltrated and difficult to distinguish from the surrounding tissue. In both models thrombocytopenia and hyperfibrinogenemia were observed, whereas microangiopathic hemolytic anemia was only seen in the 3LL model. The survival of radiolabelled fibrinogen was reduced in 3LL, whereas it was normal in JWS. Accordingly, fibrin was deposited at the tumor site in 3LL, not in JWS (4,30). Despite this difference, the fraction of cardiac output distributed per gram of tumoral tissue (measured by a radiolabelled microsphere technique) was very similar in the two tumors (33). When tested <u>in vitro</u>, 3LL cells had higher procoagulant and lower fibrinolytic activity than JWS cells (5,21). It is not known whether these properties influence the different fibrin deposition patterns observed in the two models.

PHARMACOLOGICAL MODULATION OF THE HEMOSTATIC SYSTEM
IN TUMOR-BEARING ANIMALS

Most of the information so far available on the role of platelets and coagulation in cancer growth has been derived from studies with drugs influencing the hemostatic system of tumor-bearing animals. The findings to date are highly controversial, probably because of differences in the experimental models used,

in the period of treatment during tumor growth and in a number
of other interfering factors, such as the animals' diet. Above
all, the drugs used in these studies, besides their effect on the
hemostatic system, all have a number of other pharmacological
activities which could by themselves influence cancer growth.

Different Dissemination Models

Some investigations have indicated that induction of hypo-
coagulability in animals prior to the intravenous injection of
viable tumor cells reduced the number and incidence of lung
nodule formation (19). This effect was ascribed to longer persistence of cells in the circulation in anticoagulated animals
because of better patency of the microcirculatory bed and
impairment of tumor cell-fibrin emboli formation (19,36). However, as mentioned above, the approach of mimicking blood-borne
metastases by intravenous injection of tumor cells into laboratory animals is highly artificial, since this model reflects only
the final steps of dissemination (transport in blood and take by
target organs), completely by-passing the initial phases which
include detachment from the primary tumor and entry into the
bloodstream. The clotting system may also play a role in these
initial phases. In fact, fibrin deposition around tumors may
have a dual meaning, serving both as a barrier for cancer dissemination and a preventive mechanism for the host's defences against
cancer cells, the relative importance of these effects largely
depending on the experimental conditions (9). For these and
probably many other reasons, different results have been obtained
when the same drugs were used in "spontaneous" or in "artificial"
metastasis models.

Table 3 summarizes the experience we have collected when 3LL-
bearing mice are treated with drugs influencing the host's hemostatic system at various levels. All the drugs studied (an anticoagulant, a defibrinating enzyme and two platelet aggregation
inhibitors, acetylsalicylic acid and ditazole) share some
inhibitory effect on the "artificial" metastasis model, whereas
only warfarin also markedly reduces spontaneous metastasis formation. These results are in agreement with those reported by
Hilgard (14) and illustrate the difficulty of distinguishing
which of the various steps of spontaneous dissemination is/are
controlled by anticoagulant treatment.

Table 3. Schematic representation of the effects obtained with
various drugs on artificial and spontaneous lung metastasis growth of 3LL (6,24,29).

Drug	Lung colonies	Spontaneous metastases
Warfarin	↓	↓
Batroxobin	↓	→
Aspirin	↓	→
Ditazole	↓	→

Different Phases of Growth

The effectiveness of treatment with anticoagulants or defibrinating enzymes often depends on the total length of the treatment and on the choice of appropriate periods of administration. Oral anticoagulation with warfarin, or phenprocoumon, as an example, gives the best results in terms of metastasis growth inhibition when treatment is given for the animals' whole lifespan (8,18). On the other hand, at least in the 3LL model, coumarin anticoagulation appears to affect metastasis formation more during lodgement than during detachment from the primary, since it is still active when started at day 7-10 after implantation of the 3LL cells, but it is not active if interrupted 7-10 days before the animals are killed.

A completely different picture has been obtained with defibrinating enzymes, such as batroxobin, a snake venom-derived principle.

The number of spontaneous lung metastases from JWS was reduced in mice defibrinated during the initial phase of dissemination, whereas it was unaffected in mice given batroxobin at later stages, when the lungs had already been colonized by tumor cells (3). Lung colony formation on i.v. injection of JWS cells was also reduced in defibrinated mice (3). In this experimental model, therefore, removal of the host's circulating fibrinogen appeared of benefit only during lodgement of cancer cells in the lungs at the arrest-trapping phase. This may indirectly support the contention that fibrin plays different roles in different phases of tumor growth.

Different Pharmacological Activities

The supposed antitumoral or antimetastatic activity of drugs modulating the host's hemostatic system may be influenced by a number of other factors, because of the multiplicity of the pharmacological effects of each drug. Possible modifications of cell metabolism or growth, or motility, changes in blood flow, in immune responses or in prostaglandin metabolism have all to be taken into account in assessing the impact on tumor growth of many drugs primarily used to affect the hemostatic system. As an example, controversial results have been reported so far with platelet aggregation inhibitors in experimental models of dissemination (19). Non-steroidal antiinflammatory agents have been shown to reduce tumor growth in some experimental models (22) whereas in other systems they were completely ineffective (16,24) or even increased tumor and metastasis weights (34).

It is difficult to reconcile these data, some of which have been obtained in different experimental models; but it must be recalled that these drugs act basically as inhibitors of prostaglandin synthesis, not only in platelets (where they prevent the generation of cyclic endoperoxides and thromboxanes, potent aggregating agents) but also in other cells, such as vascular

cells, macrophages and tumor cells themselves (11). Changes in
the pattern of prostaglandin generation by these cells may have
important implications on tumor growth since some PGs are responsible for immunosuppression, response to inflammatory stimuli,
anaphylactic type reactions and bone-resorbing activity of tumors
(10,22).

Cancer cells are known to produce prostaglandins mainly of the
E and F type (10); in addition, cells from two murine tumors and
their secondaries have recently been shown to generate PGI_2
(prostacyclin) (27), a potent vasodilator and modulator of blood
flow at several sites (23). In primary tissue and metastatic
nodules of both 3LL and JWS the ability to generate PGI_2 correlated well with the relative distribution of cardiac output
(measured with a labelled microsphere technique) and appeared to
modulate the tumor vasculature's response to the vasoactive agent
noradrenaline (32,33).

The production of PGI_2 by 3LL cancer cells was inhibited in
animals treated chronically with aspirin or indomethacin, but
only the latter drug was able to significantly reduce primary
tumor growth (unpublished results).

On the other hand, as discussed, snake venom enzymes have been
repeatedly used to keep animals defibrinated during growth of
experimental tumors (19). However, such agents could have other
effects potentially important for tumor growth, such as immunodepression. Indeed, both the primary humoral and the delayed
type hypersensitivity reaction were depressed in mice defibrinated
with either of two batroxobin preparations (1). This could
account at least partially for the promotion of metastatic cancer
growth observed in some experimental conditions when batroxobin
was given chronically to 3LL bearing mice (6).

As a last example, coumarin derivatives have yielded the most
consistent results in reducing primary and especially metastatic
tumor growth in rodents (7,14). However, in this case too, the
relevance of these results as an indication of the role of fibrin
in metastasis formation is questionable. Warfarin could exert a
direct cytotoxic effect or inhibit tumor cell motility and mitotic
activity (2,20).

In our experiments, the antimetastatic effect of warfarin was
closely associated with its anticoagulant activity. Experiments
using the racemic form of warfarin and each of its resolved
enantiomers showed that R-warfarin had almost no anticlotting
activity in mice and did not modify the metastatic growth of 3LL,
but the opposite was true for S-warfarin (29). However, the
observation that other anticoagulants (such as heparin) do not
share warfarin's effect (14) argues against the concept of
warfarin's antimetastatic effect being mediated only by plasma
anticoagulation.

It has recently been proposed that, in warfarin treatment,
vitamin K-dependent proteins with a γ-carboxyglutamic acid moiety
could be involved (13). The cell changes induced by vitamin K
deficiency might, however, again result in reduction of the

procoagulant activity of cancer or host cells and <u>cellular</u> anticoagulation could be important. Preliminary evidence for this effect has been obtained in the 3LL system (26).

3LL cells have a peculiar procoagulant activity (Factor X activating activity) which could contribute to the observed fibrin deposition at the tumor site in 3LL (30); this activity has been found reduced in cells harvested from tumors of animals treated chronically with warfarin at doses capable to significantly depress lung metastasis formation without affecting the primary tumor weight (Table 4).

In view of the unique antimetastatic activity of coumarin anticoagulants (7), this may indicate that, in order to achieve the control of metastasis formation, pharmacological modulation of the cell capabilities to promote local fibrin deposition is more important than general modifications of the host's hemostatic system.

Table 4. Effect of chronic treatment with warfarin on plasma prothrombin complex activity (Thrombotest) and on 3LL cell (15×10^6/ml) procoagulant activity (recalcification time). Means $\pm$ S.E. of data from 15 animals per group are reported. The warfarin schedule and the clotting tests were performed as previously described (5,29).

Experimental Group	Plasma Anticoagulation (Thrombotest) sec	Cellular Anticoagulation (Recalcification time) sec	Primary tumor (g)	Lung metastasis (mg)
Control	23.9+1.1	46.6+1.6	9.8+0.6	260+49
Warfarin (day 7-22)	> 180	81.7+2.4[**]	9.5+0.2	45+12[*]

[*] $p < 0.01$; [**] $p < 0.001$ at Student's t test

CONCLUSIONS

Findings from experimental models suggest that hemostatic changes may occur during tumor development. Evidence for a role of fibrin and/or platelets in tumor growth and metastasis is derived indirectly from pharmacological studies that are difficult to interpret.

Recent developments in the knowledge of experimental metastasis biology could provide tools for more direct evaluation of the role of fibrin in cancer cell invasiveness. Variant tumor lines have been selected with enhanced ability to form experimental pulmonary metastases in syngeneic hosts and are currently the subject of extensive investigations (31). It is hoped that the study of cell/fibrin interactions in these models with different metastatic potential will offer some more direct information on the questions raised in this review.

ACKNOWLEDGEMENTS

The authors' work mentioned in this review was performed within the frame of the "Cell-fibrin interactions" subgroup of the EORTC tumor invasion group and was partially supported by Italian National Research Council (Contract 80.01621.96), and by Grant NIH PHRB-1RO1 CA L2764-01, National Cancer Institute, NIH, Bethesda, Maryland, USA. Judith Baggott and Anna Mancini helped prepare this manuscript.

REFERENCES

1. Anaclerio, A., Ruggeri, A., Poggi, A., Spreafico F. and Donati, M.B. (1980): In vivo and in vitro immunosuppresive effect of two batroxobin preparations in mice. Thromb.Res., 18: 253-258.

2. Chang, J.C., and Hall, T.C. (1973): In vitro effect of sodium warfarin on DNA and RNA synthesis of mouse L1210 leukemic cells and Walker tumor cells. Oncology, 28: 232-237

3. Chmielewska, J., Poggi A., Janik, P., Latallo, Z.S. and Donati, M.B. (1980): Effect of defibrination with batroxobin on growth and metastasis of JW sarcoma in mice. Europ.J.Cancer, in press

4. Chmielewska, J., Poggi, A., Mussoni, L., Donati, M.B., and Garattini, S. (1980): Blood coagulation changes in JW Sarcoma, a new metastasizing tumor in mice. Eur.J.Cancer, in press

5. Curatolo, L., Colucci, M., Cambini, A.L., Poggi, A., Morasca, L., Donati, M.B., and Semeraro, N. (1979): Evidence that cells from experimental tumours can activate coagulation factor X. Br.J.Cancer, 40: 228-233.

6. Donati, M.B., Mussoni, L., Poggi, A., de Gaetano, G. and Garattini, S. (1978): Growth and metastasis of the Lewis Lung carcinoma in mice defibrinated with batroxobin. Europ.J.Cancer, 14: 343-347

7. Donati, M.B., and Poggi, A. (1980): Malignancy and Haemostasis. Brit.J.Haematol., 44: 173-182

8. Donati, M.B., Poggi, A., Mussoni, L., de Gaetano, G., and
   Garattini, S. (1977): Hemostasis and experimental cancer
   dissemination. In: Cancer Invasion and Metastasis: Biologic
   Mechanisms and Therapy, edited by S.B. Day, W.P.L. Myers,
   P. Stansly, S. Garattini, and M.G. Lewis, pp. 151-160.
   Raven Press, New York.

9. Dvorak, H.F., Dvorak, A.M., Manseau, E.J., Wiberg, L., and
   Churchill, W.H. (1979): Fibrin gel investment associated with
   line 1 and line 10 solid tumor growth, angiogenesis, and
   fibroplasia in guinea pigs. Role of cellular immunity, myo-
   fibroblasts, microvascular damage, and infarction in line 1
   tumor regression. J.Natl.Cancer Institute, 62: 1459-1472.

10. Easty, G.C., and Easty, D.M. (1976): Prostaglandins and
    Cancer. Cancer Treat.Rev., 3: 217-225

11. Flower,R.J. (1974): Drugs which inhibit prostaglandin bio-
    synthesis. Pharmacol.Rev., 26: 33-67.

12. Hilgard, P. (1973): The role of blood platelets in experi-
    mental metastases. Brit.J.Cancer, 28: 429-435

13. Hilgard, P. (1977): Experimental vitamin K deficiency and
    spontaneous metastases. Brit.J.Cancer, 35: 891-892

14. Hilgard, P.: The use of anticoagulants in tumour therapy.
    This book.

15. Hilgard, P., and Gordon-Smith, E.C. (1974): Microangiopathic
    haemolytic anaemia and experimental tumour-cell emboli.
    Brit.J.Haematol. 26: 651-659

16. Hilgard, P., Heller, H.,and Schmidt, C.G. (1976): The influ-
    ence of platelet aggregation inhibitors on metastasis forma-
    tion in mice (3LL). Z. Krebsforsch, 86: 243-250

17. Hilgard, P., Hohage, R., Schmitt, W., and Kohle, W. (1973):
    Microangiopathic haemolytic anaemia associated with hyper-
    calcaemia in an experimental rat tumour. Brit.J.Haematol.,
    24: 245-254.

18. Hilgard, P., Schulte, H., Wetzig, G., Schmitt, G., and Schmidt C.G. (1977): Oral anticoagulation in the treatment of a spontaneously metastasizing murine tumour (3LL). Brit.J. Cancer, 35: 78-85

19. Hilgard, P.,and Thornes, R.D. (1976): Anticoagulants in the treatment of cancer. Eur.J.Cancer, 12: 755-762

20. Kirsch, W.M., Schulz, D., Van Buskirk, J.J., and Young, H.E. (1974): Effects of sodium warfarin and other carcinostatic agents on malignant cells: a study of drug synergy. J.Med., 5: 69-82.

21. Latallo, Z.S., Kowalska-Loth, B., Chmielewska, J., Teisseyre, E., Raczka, E.,and Kopec, M. (1979): A new approach to study factors from tumour cells which influence the clotting and fibrinolytic systems. In: Progress in Chemical Fibrinolysis and Thrombolysis, vol. IV, edited by Davidson J.F., Cepelak V., Samama M.M., Desnoyers P.C., pp. 411-415. Churchill Livingstone, Edinburgh.

22. Lynch, N.R., Castes, M., Astoin, M., Salomon, J.C. (1978): Mechanism of inhibition of tumour growth by aspirin and indomethacin. Brit.J.Cancer, 38: 503-512

23. Moncada, S., and Vane, J.R. (1979): Arachidonic acid metabolites and the interactions between platelets and blood-vessel walls. N.Engl.J.Med., 300: 1142-1147

24. Mussoni, L., Poggi, A., de Gaetano, G., and Donati, M.B. (1978): Effect of ditazole, an inhibitor of platelet aggregation, on a metastatizing tumour in mice. Brit.J.Cancer, 37: 126-129.

25. Mussoni, L., Poggi, A., Donati, M.B., and de Gaetano, G. (1977): Ditazole and platelets. III. Effect of ditazole on tumor-cell induced thrombocytopenia and on bleeding time in mice. Haemostasis, 6: 260-265.

26. Poggi, A., Colucci, M., Delaini, F., Semeraro, N. and Donati, M.B.(1980): Reduced procoagulant activity of Lewis Lung carcinoma cells from mice treated with warfarin.

Europ.J.Cancer, in press

27. Poggi, A., Dall'Olio, A., Balconi, G., Delaini, F., de Gaetano, G., and Donati, M.B. (1979): Generation of prostacyclin (PGI_2) activity by Lewis Lung carcinoma (3LL) cells. Thromb.Haemost., 42: 339

28. Poggi, A., Donati, M.B., Polentarutti, N., de Gaetano, G.,and Garattini, S. (1976): On the thrombocytopenia developing in mice bearing a spontaneously metastasizing tumor. Z. Krebsforsch. 86: 303-306.

29. Poggi, A., Mussoni, L., Kornblihtt, L., Ballabio, E., de Gaetano, G., and Donati, M.B. (1978): Warfarin enantiomers, anticoagulation and experimental tumour metastasis. Lancet, 1: 163-164.

30. Poggi, A., Polentarutti, N., Donati, M.B., de Gaetano, G., and Garattini, S. (1977): Blood coagulation changes in mice bearing Lewis Lung carcinoma, a metastasizing tumor. Cancer Res., 37: 272-277.

31. Poste, G., and Fidler, I.J. (1980): The pathogenesis of cancer metastasis. Nature, 283: 139-146.

32. Quintana, A., Raczka, E., and Donati, M.B. (1979): Different responses to noradrenaline (NA) of vascular tissues from two metastasizing tumours in mice. Thromb.Haemostasis, 42: 140.

33. Raczka, E., Quintana, A., Poggi, A., and Donati, M.B. (1979): Cardiac output distribution in mice bearing Lewis Lung carcinoma (3LL) or JW sarcoma (JWS), two spontaneously metastasizing tumours. Thromb.Haemostasis, 42: 142

34. Santoro, M.G., Philpott, G.W., and Jaffe, B.M. (1976): Inhibition of tumour growth in vivo and in vitro by prostaglandin E. Nature, 263: 777-779.

35. Spreafico, S., and Garattini, S. (1974): Selective antimetastatic treatment. Current status and future prospects. Cancer Treat.Rev. 1, 239-250

36. White, H., and Griffiths, J.D. (1976): Circulating malignant cells and fibrinolysis during resection of colorectal cancer. Proc.Roy.Soc.Med. <u>69</u>, 467-469 (1976).

37. Yuhas, J.M., and Pazmino, N.H. (1974): Inhibition of sub- cutaneously growing line 1 carcinomas due to metastatic spread. <u>Cancer Res</u>., 34: 2005-2010

38. Zacharski, L.R., Henderson, W.G., Rickles, F.R., Forman, W.B., Cornell, C.J., Jackson Forcier, R., Harrower, H.W., and Johnson, R.O. (1979): Rationale and experimental design for the VA cooperative study of anticoagulation (warfarin) in the treatment of cancer. <u>Cancer</u>, 44: 732-741.

Malignancy and the Hemostatic System,
edited by M. B. Donati et al.
Raven Press, New York © 1981.

The Use of Oral Anticoagulants in Tumour Therapy

P. Hilgard

*Department of Haematology, Royal Postgraduate Medical School,
Hammersmith Hospital, London W12 OHS, United Kingdom*

Morphological evidence for a close association of intravascular cancer cells with thrombotic material had suggested that anticoagulants could be useful in preventing or reducing secondary tumour spread. In the rabbit ear chamber it was shown that experimental tumour cells injected into the circulation of the animal were rapidly surrounded by a fibrin-platelet thrombus which supported the fixation of the cells at the primary site of their intravascular arrest. Prevention of these thrombi around tumour emboli prolonged the circulation time of the injected cells and reduced the subsequent formation of tumour deposits (26). Numerous investigations have indicated that deceleration of blood coagulability prior to the injection of viable cancer cells into animals reduced the number and incidence of secondary tumours. Heparin, Ancrod, fibrinolytic agents, platelet aggregation inhibitors, Dextran and oral anticoagulants have been shown to possess "antimetastatic" properties in these experimental systems (9).

The approach to mimic blood borne cancer cells by injection of tumour cells into the blood stream of experimental animals is of course highly artificial and the relevance for human pathology is questionable. This criticism was met by the introduction of spontaneously metastasising, transplantable tumours as model of disease. The evaluation of the pathogenic significance of altered blood coagulability under these experimental conditions was mainly based on long-term anticoagulation of the host. It was noticed by Hagmar that Heparin anticoagulation did not influence the spontaneous metastatic spread of a methylcholanthrene-induced mouse tumour; however, under identical experimental conditions the Coumarin-derivative Phenprocoumon exerted a significant antimetastatic effect (7). In addition, Poggi et al reported that Warfarin was highly effective in reducing metastases in the Lewis Lung Carcinoma (20); in the same experimental model the authors did not find any antimetastatic effect of long-term anticoagulation with the defibrinating viper venom Batroxobin (4). These reports were confirmed by Hilgard comparing the effect of long-term Ancrod treatment with that of Coumarin anticoagulation on spontaneous metastases (11). A survey of the current literature on the effect of various anticoagulants on experimental tumour growth

and tumour spread revealed that only Coumarin-derivatives exert a
constant and significant antimetastatic effect, which appears to
be independent of the experimental tumour system under investigation. Other anticoagulants, including "antiplatelet" drugs, gave
conflicting results, and their antimetastatic action is not established. This suggests that Coumarins have a unique mode of
action which, at least in part, appears to be independent of its
effect on blood coagulability.

Table 1 shows that long-term anticoagulation of tumour bearing
mice with the Coumarin-derivative Phenprocoumon resulted in a significant decrease of the number and incidence of spontaneous lung
metastasis from the Lewis Lung Carcinoma, as well as inhibition
of primary tumour growth. The beneficial effects of Phenprocoumon were only evident when a well controlled, continuous state
of anticoagulation was achieved; deliberate interruption of therapy or short-term therapy was ineffective.

From a series of experiments with a methylcholanthrene-induced
sarcoma in mice, Hoover, Jones and Ketcham (13) concluded that
full anticoagulation in the range of 2.5 to 3 times normal is required for a maximal antimetastatic effect.

In therapeutic doses Coumarin-derivatives do not exert direct
cytotoxic effects. Pre-incubation of Lewis Lung Carcinoma cells
with Phenprocoumon prior to implantation did not alter the kinetics of tumour growth. Anticoagulation throughout the growth of
the lymphoid leukaemia L1210 in DBA/2 mice did not influence the
mean survival time of these animals (10), and short-term Warfarin
therapy was ineffective on primary or metastatic L1210 leukaemia,
and adenocarcinoma 755 (8). On the other hand, however, high doses of Warfarin led to an inhibition of thymidine and uridine uptake into the DNA and RNA of L1210 leukaemia cells (2), and Warfarin suspended cell replication of malignant human glial cells
in culture even at low concentrations (14). Furthermore, in vivo
anticoagulation with Warfarin selectively inhibited cancer cell
motility in the rabbit ear chamber, and this effect could be reversed by the administration of vitamin K (24). From the fore-
going it thus appears that, although not having a major cytotoxic
effect, Warfarin indirectly interferes with certain cellular
functions.

Table 1.   Effect of Various Treatment Schedules on Tumour Parameters

	Mean tumour weight on day 20 (% of control group)	Mean number of lung metastases on day 20 (% of control group)	% animals with lung metastases
Control	-	-	100
Continuous phen[1] (day 1-11)	89 (n.s.)[2]	92 (n.s.)[2]	98 (n.s.)[2]
Continuous phen[1] (day 1-20)	68 ($p < 0.05$)[3]	8.6 ($p < 0.001$)[3]	51 ($p < 0.001$)[3]
Intermittent phen[1] (day 1-11)	102 (n.s.)[2]	98 (n.s.)[2]	100 (n.s.)[2]
Intermittent phen[1] (day 1-20)	76 ($p = 0.05$)[3]	112 (n.s.)[2]	100 (n.s.)[2]

1. phen = phenprocoumon

2. n.s. = not significant

3. Significance established by U-test (Wilcoxon, Mann & Whitney)

Table 2.   Treatment Haemostatically Effective at Time
of i.v. Tumour Cell Challenge (LL)

Treatment	No. of Animals	% Lung Colonies of Control	Significance
Heparin (s.c.)	20	6	$p < 0.01$[2]
Warfarin (oral)	24	3	$p < 0.01$[2]
Ancrod (s.c.)	20	12	$p < 0.01$[2]
Aspirin (i.p. + oral)	25	121	n.S.[1]
RA 233 (i.p.)	25	118	n.S.[1]

[1] n.S = not significant

[2] Significance established by U-test (Wilcoxon, Mann & Whitney)

Table 2 shows that various anticoagulants reduced the incidence
of lung colonies when anticoagulation was effectively established
at the time of i.v. challenge with Lewis Lung Carcinoma cells.
When the drugs are administered 24 hours after cell injection,
only Warfarin reduced the subsequent development of lung tumour
deposits (Table 3).

This finding suggests that Warfarin acts on metastatic tumour
growth predominantly after the initial intravascular arrest of
the malignant cells. The anticoagulant effect during the initial phase of tumour cell lodgment is apparently of minor importance since restoration of blood coagulability with human prothrombin complex before tumour cell challenge did not abolish the
antimetastatic effect of Coumarin anticoagulation (12).

Diet-induced vitamin K deficiency is as effective as Coumarin
anticoagulation in reducing tumour colonies, supporting the view
that the antimetastatic action of Coumarins is not a primary drug
effect (12). As mentioned above, clotting factor abnormalities
probably play only a minor part in the effect of oral anticoagulants on tumour growth and tumour spread. Therefore, it is likely that alterations of the vitamin K metabolism are of some importance through hitherto unrecognized mechanisms. Hypothetically

Table 3.   Treatment Initiated 24 Hours After
                  I.V. Tumour Cell Challenge (LL)

Treatment	No. of Animals	% Lung Colonies of Control	Significance
Heparin (s.c.)	12	98	n.s.[1]
Warfarin (oral)	15	7	P 0.01[2]
Ancrod (s.c.)	12	109	n.s.[1]
Aspirin (i.p. + oral)	14	104	n.s.[1]

[1] n.s. = not significant

[2] Significance established by U-test (Wilcoxon, Mann & Whitney)

the reduction of γ-carboxyglutamic acid residues on certain proteins could lead to significant effects on cell membranes through the reduction of calcium and phospholipid binding sites (23).

Macrophages play an important role in controlling tumour growth and tumour spread, and they appear to represent the target cell for non-specific immunostimulants, which under certain experimental circumstances, can reduce or inhibit metastatic tumour spread (1). Fig. 1 shows the phagocytic index of peritoneal macrophages of control and Phenprocoumon anticoagulated mice with and without non-specific immunostimulation. It is evident that anticoagulation alone did not activate macrophages; it enhances however, their activity when they are stimulated by thioglycollate or corynebacterium parvum. This effect of Coumarin anticoagulants might be of relevance to the antimetastatic action of these drugs. This is further supported by Maat's finding that macrophage inhibitors such as Silica and Carrageenan abolish the antimetastatic effect of Warfarin in the Lewis Lung Carcinoma, and in the B16 Melanoma of mice (18).

Tumour cells and tumour cell lines synthesize a clot promoting enzyme with Factor X activating activity (22), and it was suggested that this thromboplastic activity was of significance for the metastatic capacity of tumours (15). Long-term anticoagulation with Phenprocoumon considerably reduced the clot promoting activity, in particular the Factor X activating enzyme of the Lewis Lung Carcinoma, whereas, anticoagulation did not affect the tissue thromboplastin activity of muscle extracts (Table 4).

Figure 1. Phagocytic indices of peritoneal macrophages derived C57BL mice treated in vivo for 6 days with Phenprocoumon (phen) and/or a single dose of non-specific immunostimulants. 1 = control (no treatment), 2 = phen, 3 = control + thioglycollate (i.p.), 4 = phen + thioglycollate (i.p.), 5 = control + corynebacterium parvum (i.v.), 6 = phen + corynebacterium parvum (i.v.).

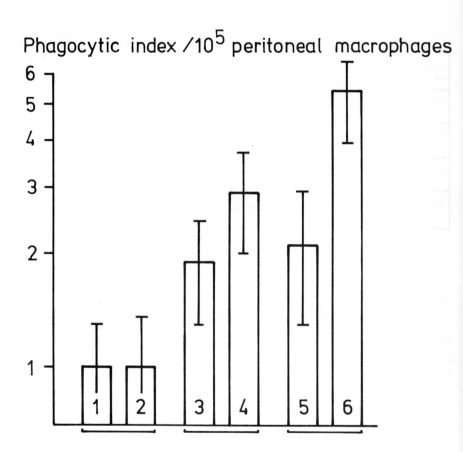

Phagocytic index /10^5 peritoneal macrophages

Table 4.   Clot Promoting Activity of Various
Tissue Extracts

Thromboplastin Activity*

	F X activating activity (Substrate: F VII def. plasma)	Tissue factor activity (Substrate: normal plasma)
Standard brain thromboplastin (n=22)	82 sec (range:78-83)	14 sec (range:13-15)
Control muscle (n=5)	82 sec (range:73-92)	18 sec (range:15-21)
Warfarin muscle (n=3)	84 sec (range:79-89)	20 sec (range:18-21)
Control tumour**(n=5)	28 sec (range:24-32)	24 sec (range:18-26)
Warfarin tumour**(n=5)	48 sec (range:39-54)	35 sec (range:28-42)

* Assay: 0.1 ml tissue extract (Protein content: 20g/l)
    + 0.1 0.025M $CaCl_2$ + substrate plasma
    clotting time recorded.

** Lewis Lung Carcinoma, 14 days after i.m. transplantation.

This finding may also have implications for the growth and spread of malignant tumours, and it provides an additional explanation for the therapeutic effect of Coumarin-derivatives on tumour metastases.

Experimentally the anti-tumour effect of oral anticoagulants can be further exploited by adding them to other therapeutic approaches. As outlined above, there is a definite role for the combination of these anticoagulants with immunotherapy. Clinical evidence suggests that the results of irradiation might be improved by concomitant anticoagulation therapy (17). In particular, the reduction of toxicity of radiotherapy by Warfarin anticoagulation warrants further consideration (16). Experimental evidence to support the clinical data is as yet conflicting (5, 21). Long-term anticoagulation with Coumarin compounds appeared to enhance the effect of some cytotoxic drugs by additive anti-tumour action; drug synergy may however, also occur(10).

It was shown that Warfarin may act synergistically with 5-Fluor-ouracil by altering the tissue distribution and plasma clearance of the drug (14). In tissue culture a unique interaction between Warfarin and Adriamycin was recently demonstrated (3), which, substantiated, could have significant therapeutic implications.

In summary, sufficient evidence indicates that oral anticoagulants of the Coumarin type interfere with malignant cell proliferation, but the exact mode of action remains to be established. In this context it is important to consider the complex pharmacology of the oral anticoagulants. In 1945 Goth was the first investigator to show that Coumarins inhibit the growth of bacteria (6), and subsequent studies suggested an important role of vitamin K in cell metabolism through its participation in mitochondrial oxidative phosphorylation (19). The discovery of the biochemical background of the role of vitamin K in protein synthesis has opened a new field of research and it has become evident that vitamin K no longer is the unique coagulation vitamin, but that it is required for the synthesis of many hitherto unknown protein structures (23). Scarce clinical evidence clearly indicated that interference with vitamin K physiology through Coumarin anticoagulants also alters the course of human malignant diseases (25, 27). Priority should be given to further clinical trials in order to learn more about the possible role of Coumarin anticoagulants in cancer therapy.

ACKNOWLEDGMENT

Parts of the author's experimental work were supported by grants from the "Deutsche Forschungsgemeinschaft", Bad-Godesberg, FRG (Hi 213/2-4).

REFERENCES

1. Alexander, P., Eccles, S.A. and Gauci, C.L.L. (1976): Ann. N.Y. Acad. Sci., 276:124
2. Chang, J.C. and Hall, T.C. (1973): Oncology, 28:232
3. Dolfini, E., Ghersa, P., Barbieri, B., Donelli, M.G. and Fuhrman Conti, A.M. (1979): in Press.
4. Donati, M.B., Mussoni, L., Poggi, A., de Gaetano, G. and Garattini, S. (1978): Europ. J. Cancer, 14:343.
5. Frischkorn, R., Rath, W., and Doench, K. (1976): Strahlentherapie, 151:214.
6. Goth, A. (1945): Science, 101:383.
7. Hagmar, B. (1968): Path. europ., 3:622.
8. Higashi, H. and Heidelberger, C. (1971): Cancer Chemother. Rep. Part 1, 55:29.
9. Hilgard, P. and Thornes, R.D. (1976): Europ. J. Cancer, 12:755.
10. Hilgard, P., Schulte, H., Wetzig, G., Schmitt, G. and Schmidt, C.G. (1977): Brit. J. Cancer, 35:78.
11. Hilgard, P. (1977): Brit. J. Cancer, 35 891.
12. Hilgard, P. and Maat, B. (1979): Europ J. Cancer, 15 183.
13. Hoover, H.C., Jones, D. and Ketcham, A.S. (1976): Surgery, 79:625.
14. Kirsch, W.M., Schulz, D., van Buskirk, J.J. and Young, H.E. (1974): J. Med., 5:69.
15. Koike, A. (1964): Cancer, 17:450.
16. Lightdale, C.J., Wasser, J., Coleman, M., Brower, M., Teft, M., and Pasmantier, M. (1979): Cancer, 43:174.
17. Ludwig, H. (1974): Gyakologe, 7:1.
18. Maat, B. (1978): Annual Report of the Radiobiological Institute TNO, Rijswijk, The Netherlands.
19. Martius, C. and Nitz-Litzow, D. (1953): Biochim. biophys. Acta 12:134.
20. Poggi, A., Mussoni, L., Kornblihtt, L., Ballabio, E., de Gaetano, G. and Donati, M.B. (1978): Lancet, i:163.
21. Rottinger, E.M., Sedlacek, R., Suit, H.D. (1975): Europ. J. Cancer, 11:743.
22. Semeraro, N. (1979): Thrombos. Haemostas., (Stuttg.),42:352.
23. Stenflo, J. and Suttie, J.W. (1977): Ann. Reu. Biochem., 46:157.
24. Thornes, R.D., Edlow, D.W. and Wood Jr., S. (1968): John Hopk. med. J., 123:305.
25. Thornes, R.D. (1975): Cancer, 35:91.
26. Wood Jr., S. (1974): J. Med., 5:7.
27. Zacharski, L.R. (1979): Thrombos. Haemostas. (Stuttg.), 42:353.

Malignancy and the Hemostatic System,
edited by M. B. Donati et al.
Raven Press, New York © 1981.

Anticoagulation in the Treatment of Cancer in Man

Leo R. Zacharski

*Dartmouth Medical School, Veterans Administration Hospital,
White River Junction, Vermont 05001*

INTRODUCTION

There is now little doubt that the coagulation mechanism is involved in the pathogenesis of human malignancy. Over a century ago, Billroth[1] noted thrombi in association with microscopic intravascular tumor deposits. He postulated that embolization of tumor bearing thrombi was responsible for metastasis formation. This microanatomic association between tumor cells and elements of clotted blood has been reaffirmed on a number of occasions since that time[2-8]. The observation of tumor cells in mitosis within thrombi in several of these studies[3-5] led to the hypothesis that such an environment provided a suitable "culture medium" for tumor growth. These histopathologic studies were succeeded by additional studies in which various histochemical stains[9-10] as well as immunologic and radioisotopic labelling procedures[11-16] were used to demonstrate the existence of the two structural elements of clots, namely fibrin and platelets, in association with tumors.

Activation of the coagulation mechanism can occur not only at tumor sites but also within the systemic circulation. Such activation is recognizable in the form of localized thromboembolic events or as disseminated intravascular coagulation (DIC). The association of malignancy with thromboembolic disease has been recognized for over a hundred years and has been reviewed by Sack and co-workers[17]. Recently, a significantly increased incidence of thromboembolic events has been confirmed in cancer patients in contrast to patients without neoplastic disease[18]. DIC is frequently detectable because of attendant coagulation test abnormalities[18-19].

The mechanism by which elements of clots are deposited at tumor sites is not entirely clear. However, a coagulant extractable from tumor tissue may be responsible. While controversy remains as to the precise nature of this coagulant[20-23], it has

been identified as tissue factor (tissue thromboplastin) in
certain types of malignant cells[24-26]. Conceivably, more than one
coagulant and/or fibrinolytic enzyme is operative in various malignancies or even in a single malignancy.

Should an intact coagulation mechanism be required for the
growth and spread of malignancy, one might expect to see a reduced incidence of or death rate from cancer in individuals with
hereditary coagulation disorders or in individuals previously
treated with anticoagulants. Forman[27] studied the occurrence of
cancer in individuals with bleeding disorders. From a total of
10,500 such individuals identified by postal survey, he found 61
with malignancy. A reduced incidence of or death rate from malignancy, as compared to an appropriate control population, was not
found. In fact, there seemed to be an excess of patients with
soft tissue sarcomas. However, the paucity of individuals in this
series with deficiencies of factor II, V, VII and X, and of individuals with platelet disorders may make a study of this type an
inadequate test of this relationship. This is because of the
likelihood that malignant cells initiate clot formation by way of
the so-called extrinsic pathway of blood coagulation[28] and this
pathway requires the presence of these factors[29].

Other clues to a possible relationship between the coagulation
mechanism and malignancy might be obtained by studying the morbid-
ity and mortality from cancer in previously anticoagulated individuals. Such a study has been performed by Michaels[30-31]. 540
patients who received anticoagulant therapy for at least three
months for thrombolic disease during the years 1951 - 1963 were
followed a total of 1,569 person-years while they were on anticoagulant treatment. During the follow-up period, there were 10
cases of cancer while the expected number, based on tumor registry
data, was 11. Although the incidence of malignancy was therefore
that which was expected, the author reported a significantly
reduced cancer mortality since there was only one death from
cancer while the expected number was 7.9. It is not known, however, how many patients were withdrawn from anticoagulant therapy
once the diagnosis of cancer was made. Such individuals would,
therefore, contribute to the incidence of but not the mortality
from malignancy since they would have died of malignancy after
anticoagulant therapy had been discontinued. This issue remains
unsettled.

CLINICAL TRIALS OF ANTICOAGULANTS IN CANCER

Undoubtedly the best test of the relationship between the coagulation mechanism and the growth and spread of malignancy would
be to determine the consequences of anticoagulant administration
to patients with malignancy. Within a decade of the first successful use of anticoagulants in ameliorating tumors in experimental animals[32], such clinical trials of anticoagulants in human

malignancy were, in fact, begun. Between 1961 and 1967, Thornes initiated studies of warfarin in patients with advanced malignancy [33-37]. In his first study of 96 patients[33], the relative safety of such treatment was described and 26 of these were thought to have responded. Subsequently, he studied a series of 30 additional patients similarly treated and found that patients with Hodgkins' disease and chronic myeloid leukemia required lower doses of maintenance chemotherapy when also treated with warfarin[36]. 128 patients with a variety of advanced cancers were then studied in a systematic fashion[35-36]. Every other patient with the same histologic type was given warfarin in addition to conventional therapy which was given to all patients. The 2-year survival was significantly greater in the warfarin group (40.6%) than in the control group (17.8%). It was Thornes' impression that ovarian and breast cancer, and lymphosarcomas might be particularly responsive to the addition of warfarin to conventional therapy. Thornes emphasized the need to administer warfarin continuously and on a long-term basis[35]. Also reported were preliminary data on the use of fibrinolytic therapy following resection for colon cancer[37]. Results presented in this and a separate paper[38] were judged to be promising but inconclusive due to lack of complete follow up. In another report, evidence was presented that fibrinolytic therapy reversed anergy which is commonly a feature of patients with advanced cancer[39].

More recently, 44 patients with advanced breast cancer were studied by the same group[40]. Half of these were treated with conventional chemotherapy and half with the same therapy together with BCG, plus levamisol and warfarin. A 17 month median survival was noted in the former group and a 34 month survival in the latter.

Anticoagulants have been administered to a number of patients with carcinoma of the lung[33,35,41-50]. In pilot studies, Elias and associates[42,43] showed in a small number of patients that heparin anticoagulation, while having no apparent tumor inhibitory effect of its own, potentiated the ability of cytotoxic drugs to induce tumor regression. Subsequently this group reported that administration of heparin together with combination chemotherapy was associated with regression of advanced cancer in 7 of 14 cases [44]. No regressions were noted in 14 historical control patients treated similarly but without heparin.

In an attempt to confirm these results, Edlis and co-workers[45] treated 19 advanced lung cancer patients with a combination of heparin and chemotherapy and noted only a single instance of tumor regression. Rohwedder and Sagastume[46] treated 16 patients in a similar manner and described a partial response in only 3. Thus, these authors were unable to confirm the earlier findings of Elias et al[44]. They concluded that anticoagulation had little effect.

A notable difference between the former study and the latter two studies might explain the divergent findings. In the earlier study of Elias et al[44], 5 of the 14 patients in the experimental group had large cell undifferentiated carcinoma[47] and 4 of these 5 were among the 7 that achieved tumor regression. Six of the 14 patients in the control group (that did not receive heparin) had a large cell undifferentiated cell type and none of these responded. By contrast, undifferentiated carcinoma was the cell type in only 3 of the 19 patients reported by Edlis et al[45] and in none of the 16 patients reported by Rohwedder and Sagastume[46]. Therefore, the difference in responsiveness upon addition of heparin to combination chemotherapy could have been a reflection of an imbalance in the cell types represented. The effect of anticoagulation on longevity was not investigated in any of these studies.

In a recently reported study by Stanford[48], 24 patients with small cell carcinoma of the lung were randomly allocated to receive chemotherapy with or without anticoagulants. Anticoagulation was accomplished with intermittent intravenous heparin and dextran, and oral warfarin was administered between courses. No difference was observed in median survival between the groups.

Salsali and Cliffton[49] reported on their experience with the treatment of malignant obstruction of the superior vena cava. For 12 patients treated with fibrinolytic therapy plus radiation, the median survival was 12.8 months and the longest survival 6 years. Complete relief of caval obstruction was observed in 5 of the 12 cases. Comparison was made with patients treated with radiation therapy alone. For these, the median survival was 8.4 months and the longest survival 36 months. These authors claimed that with fibrinolytic therapy, clinical improvement was more rapid, recanalization more complete and survival improved. In a subsequent report[50], these authors reported that one of the patients treated with fibrinolytic therapy had had histologically proven malignancy but died 4 years and 10 months after treatment. No residual malignancy was evident at postmortem examination.

Hoover and associates[51] studied the effect of warfarin anticoagulation on the course of osteogenic sarcoma. Warfarin therapy was initiated 7 days prior to surgery and then continued during the procedure (amputation) and for six months thereafter. While comparison was made with historical controls and relatively small numbers of cases were studied, survival was thought to be significantly increased in the anticoagulated group.

In other studies, several patients with malignant melanoma[52] were treated with fibrinolytic agents with equivocal results. Larsen and colleagues[41] treated 11 patients with various advanced malignancies with intermittant infusions of porcine plasmin over periods of time from 2 weeks to 8 months. Each patient also received oral aspirin and intravenous heparin with each plasmin infusion. Apparently no cancer chemotherapy or radiation therapy was used. Objective tumor regression was claimed in 4 of these cases, 2 of whom had lung cancer, one stomach cancer and one metastatic cancer of unknown primary site. Williams and Maugham[53] reported regression of colon, lung and breast tumors upon initiation of Ancrod therapy which induces hypofibrinogenemia. Patients with carcinoma of the pancreas treated by Waddell[54] with 5-fluorouracil plus warfarin were said to live "slightly longer" than patients who received other forms of treatment or who were untreated. O'Halloran and O'Meara[55] described "certain favorable, short-term observations" in 10 patients with advanced carcinoma of the breast treated with protamine.

A retrospective study of patients with stage II and III carcinoma of the cervix was reported by Reis and associates[56]. They reasoned that an effect of anticoagulation on the course of this malignancy might be observable among these patients since some were treated with anticoagulants (heparin and warfarin) at the time they received conventional therapy in order to prevent thromboembolic complications. Analysis revealed 1,393 who received conventional treatment but no anticoagulant. Among these, the recurrence rate was 22.9% after 5 to 8 months followup. By contrast, in 1,674 patients who were similarly treated but who received prophylactic anticoagulation, the recurrence rate was 12.6%. Survival was also said to be increased in the anticoagulated group but the statistical significance of the difference was not given. These workers also reported the occurrence of fibrin in tumor sections on histopathologic examination of non-anticoagulated subjects. This fibrin was decreased or absent in tumors from individuals treated with anticoagulants.

A well-studied case of papillary adenocarcinoma of the ovary was reported by Astedt and associates[57]. Reduction in malignant ascites was observed following radiation therapy together with progestogen, cyclophosphamide, heparin and the fibrinolytic inhibitor tranexamic acid. Progression of disease was noted following cessation of therapy. However, resumption of heparin and tranexamic acid without other therapy was once again followed by regression. Laparotomy was performed at the time of diagnosis and again subsequent to all of the above therapy. Little tumor progression was evident. Remarkably, histologic examination revealed a dense fibrin encasement of nests of tumor cells following treatment which was not evident before treatment. These authors postulated that the histologic change and possibly the apparent clinical benefit were related to the tranexamic acid and that the heparin contributed little to the result.

Astedt and associates[58] also reported a case of advanced breast cancer having bone, brain and pleural metastases, that had become refractory to conventional chemotherapy and radiation therapy. Treatment was then begun with twice-daily subcutaneous heparin plus oral tranexamic acid to inhibit fibrinolysis. The pleural effusion subsequently disappeared and the previously abnormal brain scan became normal. The patient was judged to be free of disease 18 months after detection of cerebral metastases. Similar benefit was claimed by the authors for mesothelioma and ovarian carcinoma but details were not presented.

Kirsch and co-workers[59] reported their experience in treating over 120 patients with inoperable tumors of the central nervous system. Treatment included anticoagulation with warfarin, radiation therapy and several chemotherapeutic agents. A favorable response was claimed for some of these and two patients with thalamic glioblastomas lived 2.5 years. A 10 month median survival was described in ten patients with multiple intracranial metastases. This was contrasted with the 2 to 3 months that these authors would have expected.

White and Griffiths[60] reviewed evidence obtained from experimental tumor systems which indicated that persistence of tumor cells within the circulation is associated with a reduced number of tumor takes. The implication was that tumor cells must adhere in order to survive and that non-adherent cells continue to circulate and ultimately die. With this background, they studied circulating tumor cells in patients with Duke's A, B and C carcinoma of the colon both during and at intervals after resection. They showed that patients in whom circulating tumor cells were demonstrable had an improved 10 year survival in contrast to patients in which such cells were not demonstrable. They also found in 50 patients that circulating tumor cells were invariably gone by one hour after surgery. These workers then studied 5 patients to whom urokinase was administered immediately upon removal of the tumor. In each case, persistence of circulating tumor cells was observed for up to 5 hours. These authors suggested that their findings provided a basis for the hypothesis that administration of fibrinolytic enzymes might forestall recurrence and prolong survival in carcinoma of the colon.

Several patients with leukemia have been treated with a fibrinolytic agent with or without warfarin[61-64]. Remission or improvement was observed in some of these. Drapkin et al[65], presented evidence that patients with acute promyelocytic leukemia were more likely to achieve remission when treated with heparin at the time they received their initial chemotherapy. This beneficial effect was thought to be due to amelioration of DIC (with resulting reduction of hemorrhagic complications) which is frequently precipitated by chemotherapy. It is of interest that the fibrinolytic inhibitor epsilon aminocaproic acid has also been administered therapeutically to patients with leukemia (as well as other malignant and nonmalignant conditions)[66]. However, the intent was to control bleeding thought due to excessive fibrinolysis and consideration was not given to the effect of this agent on the course of the primary disease.

DISCUSSION

A substantial literature exists on the effects of anticoagulants in experimental tumor systems[67-71] and on the therapeutic administration of anticoagulants to patients with malignancy[72,73]. However this approach to cancer management has not been widely accepted. The most likely explanation for this lack of acceptance is the fact that virtually all of these clinical studies have been either uncontrolled or poorly controlled. For example, well known difficulties in interpretation arise when historical controls are used and when uncertainty exists as to whether experimental and control groups are properly matched. They are therefore unconvincing since they are little more than anecdotal.

These clinical studies manifest other deficiencies as well. For example, the precise cell type of tumors under investigation is often not specified. In addition, the use of various therapeutic modalities in combination has sometimes precluded definition of the effects of single agents. This is of substantial theoretical importance since the mechanism of action of the various coagulation-inhibitory agents may be quite different. There are at least 4 mechanisms by which these agents might exert their effect[67-73]: 1) Fibrin formation at the tumor periphery may be inhibited. This fibrin may exert a protective effect against host defense mechanisms. Alternatively, fibrin may serve as a lattice upon which the cells can grow. This would be analogous to the enhancement of proliferation of cells when cultured *in vitro* in the presence of a fibrin clot[74]. 2) Warfarin might reduce tumor cell tissue factor (thromboplastin) directly[75], thereby effecting a reduction in local coagulation. 3) Warfarin (an other agents) may have direct cytotoxic effects which result, for example, in reduced cell motility[71,76,77]. 4) These agents may potentiate immunologic anti-tumor mechanisms[39,78,79] or the cytotoxic effects of conventional chemotherapeutic agents[80-82]. Standard chemotherapy protocols usually do not take into consideration whether or not anticoagulants are administered simultaneously, for example, to prevent thrombosis at the site of an intravenous catheter. At present, there is little basis for choice between these possibilities.

It is also conceivable that some agents which modify coagulation reactions may actually enhance tumor spread while others exert an inhibitory effect[83]. For example, seemingly subtle differences in the coagulative and/or fibrinolytic properties of experimental neoplastic cell lines which are similar or identical in other respects[84] may account for whether a given tumor is influenced by a given anticoagulant or antifibrinolytic agent. While these relationships are obviously complex, they may not be trivial. Coagulative and fibrinolytic enzymes are constituents of the cell periphery and thus are capable of modifying the local environment of the cell. Conceivably, such modification might explain how the neoplastic cell gains a competitive advantage over the host such that its survival and growth is ensured[85].

From this point of view, modulation of these reactions therapeutically would serve to enhance host responsiveness to the tumor and would be analagous to immunotherapy but would be distinct from conventional chemotherapy. For the latter, the toxic effect is hopefully greater toward the tumor than toward the host, but this is unfortunately not always the case. Unfortunately no means is currently available for predicting which coagulation-modifying agent or agents, if any, a given tumor will respond to.

In my view, an adequate basis now exists for carefully controlled trials of agents which modify coagulation reactions in human malignancy. Although the extent to which studies in experimental tumor systems can be applied to human tumors is unknown, such studies have frequently shown clear-cut efficacy. Some of the investigations accomplished thus far in humans have also been promising despite their many shortcomings. A variety of therapeutic agents, of which the pharmacology and toxicity are quite well defined, are available for testing. These include heparin, warfarin, platelet-inhibitory drugs (such as aspirin and dipyridamole), fibrinolytic agents (such as urokinase and streptokinase), as well as fibrinolytic inhibitors (such as epsilon aminocaproic acid and trasylol). In addition, a number of laboratory tests are available which can be used to study the hypercoagulable state in cancer patients as well as to monitor various forms of therapy in order to assess their efficacy in modifying coagulation reactions and to ensure their safe administration.

The same systematic approach that is used for evaluating conventional cancer chemotherapeutic agents is required for evaluating agents which modify coagulation reactions[86]. At this early stage, this would best be accomplished by carefully controlled prospective trials of single agents in specific tumor catagories. A VA cooperative study was initiated in 1976 and is now in progress using this approach[73]. Warfarin is the particular agent under investigation. Similar studies designed in the future should consider not only the effect of these agents on tumor regression but also their effect on longevity since anticoagulants may have their main effect on tumor spread rather than the primary tumor. Trials are justified in the presence of extensive as well as limited disease. Should positive results be forthcoming, benefit might be accrued not only in terms of patient care but also in terms of fundamental knowledge concerning the nature of neoplasia.

REFERENCES

1. Billroth, T.: Lectures on Surgical Pathology and Therapeutics, translated from the 8th Ed., the New Sydenham Society, London, 1878.

2. Schmidt, M.D.: Die verbreitungswege der karzinome und die beziehung generalisierter sarkome zu den leukamischen neubildungen. Gustav Fisher, Jena, 1903.

3. Iwasaki, T.: Histological and experimental observations on the destruction of tumor cells in the blood vessels. J Path Bacteriol 20:85-104, 1915.

4. Willis, R.A.: The Spread of Tumours in the Human Body. J and A. Churchill, London, 1934.

5. Saphir, O.: The fate of carcinoma emboli in the lung. Am J Pathol 23:245-253, 1947.

6. Morgan, A.D.: The pathology of subacute cor pulmonale in diffuse carcinomatosis of the lungs. J Path Bact 61:75-84, 1949.

7. Durham, J.R., Ashley, P.F. and Corencamp, D.: Cor pulmonale due to tumor emboli. Review of literature and report of a case. JAMA 175:757, 1961.

8. Winterbauer, R.H., Elfenbein, I.B. and Ball, W.C., Jr.: Incidence and clinical significance of tumor embolization to the lungs. Am J Med 45:271-290, 1968.

9. O'Meara, R.A.Q. and Jackson, R.D.: Cytological observations on carcinoma. Irish J Med Sci 6:327-328, 1959.

10. O'Meara, R.A.Q.: Fibrin formation and tumour growth. Thrombos Diath Haemorrh (Suppl) 28:137-142, 1968.

11. Agostino, D.: Enhancement of pulmonary metastasis following intravenous infusion of a suspension of ellagic acid. Tumori 56:29, 1970.

12. Marrack, D., Kubala, M., Corry, P., Leavens, M., Howze, J., Dewey, W., Bale, W.F. and Spar, I.L.: Localization of intracranial tumors. Comparative study with ^{131}I-labeled antibody to human fibrinogen and neohydrin [203]Hg. Cancer 20: 751-755, 1967.

13. McCardle, R.J., Harper, P.V., Spar, I.L., Bale, W.F., Andros, G. and Jiminez, F.: Studies with iodine-131-labeled antibody to human fibrinogen for diagnosis and therapy of tumors. J Nuclear Med 7:837-847, 1966.

14. Spar, I.L., Bale, W.F., Goodland, R.L., DiChiro, G.: Preparation of purified I^{131} labeled antisera to human fibrinogen. Preliminary studies in tumor patients. Acta Un Int Cancer 19:197-200, 1963.

15. Strauli, P.: Intravascular clotting and cancer localization. Diath Haemorrh (Suppl) 20:147-160, 1965.

16. Hiramoto, R., Bernecky, J., Jurandowski, J. and Pressman, D.: Fibrin in human tumors. Cancer Res 20:592-593, 1960.

17. Sack, G.H., Jr., Levin, J., Bell, W.R.: Trusseau's syndrome and other manifestations of chronic disseminated coagulopathy in patients with neoplasms: clinical, pathophysiologic and therapeutic features. Medicine 56:1-37, 1977.

18. Ambrus, J.L., Ambrus, C.M., Pickern, J., Solder, S. and Bross, I.: Hematologic changes and thromboembolic complications in neoplastic disease and their relationship to metastasis. J Med 6:433-458, 1975.

19. Owen, C.A., Jr. and Bowie, E.J.W. (editors): Symposium on The Intravascular Coagulation-Fibrinolysis (ICF) Syndromes. Mayo Clin Proc 49:627-698, 1974.

20. O'Meara, R.A.Q.: Coagulative properties of cancers. Irish J Med Sci 6:474-479, 1958.

21. Pineo, G.F., Regoeczi, E., Hatton, M.W.C. and Brain, M.C.: The activation of coagulation by extracts of mucus: a possible pathway of intravascular coagulation accompanying adenocarcinomas. J Lab Clin Med 82:255-266, 1973.

22. Pineo, G.F., Brain, M.C., Gallus, A.S., Hirsh, J., Hatton, M.W.C. and Rogoeczi, E.: Tumors, mucus production and hypercoagulability. Ann NY Acad Sci 230:262-270, 1974.

23. Gordon, S.G., Franks, J.J., Lewis, B.: Cancer procoagulant A: a factor X activating procoagulant from malignant tissue. Thrombos Res 6:127-137, 1975.

24. Gouault-Heilmann, M., Chardon, E., Sultan, C. and Josso, F.: The procoagulant factor of leukaemic promyelocytes: demonstration of immunologic cross-reactivity with human brain tissue factor. Br J Haematol 30:151-158, 1975.

25. Gralnick, H.R. and Abrell, E.: Studies of the procoagulant and fibrinolytic activity of promyelocytes in acute promyelocytic leukemia. Br J Haematol 24:89-99, 1973.

26. Sakuragawa, N., Takahashi, K., Hoshiyama, M., Jimbo, C., Matsuoka, M. and Yashikisa, O.: Pathologic cells as procoagulant substance of disseminated intravascular coagulation syndrome in acute promyelocytic leukemia. Thrombos Res 8: 263-273, 1976.

27. Forman, W.B.: Cancer in persons with congenital bleeding disorders. Cancer, in press, 1979.

28. Gralnick, H.R., Tan, H.K.: Acute promyelocytic leukemia. A model for understanding the role of the malignant cell in hemostasis. Human Path 5:661-673, 1974.

29. Nemerson, Y. and Pitlick, F.A.: The tissue factor pathway of blood coagulation, in Progress in Hemostasis and Thrombosis, Vol. 1, Spaet, T.H. (ed.), Grune and Stratton, New York, 1972, pp. 1-37.

30. Michaels, L.: Cancer incidence and mortality in patients having coagulant therapy. Lancet 2:832, 1964.

31. Michaels, L.: The incidence and course of cancer in patients receiving anticoagulant therapy. J Med 5:98-105, 1974.

32. Terranova, T. and Chiossoni, F.: Il fattore coagulazione nell'attecchimento delle cellule neoplastiche immesse in circulo. Boll Soc ital Biol sper 28:1224-1225, 1952.

33. Thornes, R.D.: Anticoagulant therapy in patients with cancer. J Irish Med Assoc 62:426-429, 1969.

34. Thornes, R.D.: Fibrin and cancer. Brit Med J 1:110, 1972.

35. Thornes, R.D.: Warfarin as maintenance therapy for cancer. J Irish Coll Phys Surg 2:41-42, 1972.

36. Thornes, R.D.: Oral anticoagulant therapy of human cancer. J Med 5:83-91, 1974.

37. Thornes, R.D.: Adjuvant therapy of cancer via the cellular immune mechanism or fibrin by induced fibrinolysis and oral anticoagulants. Cancer 35:91-97, 1975.

38. Clery, A.P., Hogan, B.L., Holland, P.D.J., Widdess, J.D.H., Ryan, M., Doyle, J.S., Burke, G.J. and Thornes, R.D.: Early experience in a controlled clinical trial using streptokinase induced fibrinolysis during resections for colon and rectal carcinomas in an attempt to prevent hematogenous metastasis. J Irish Coll Phys Surg 1:91-95, 1972.

39. Thornes, R.D.: Unblocking or activation of cellular immune mechanism by induced proteolysis in patients with cancer. Lancet 2:382-384, 1974.

40. D'Souza, D., Daly, L., and Thornes, R.D.: Levamisole, BCG and warfarin as adjuvants to chemotherapy for increased survival in advanced breast cancer. Irish Med J 71:605-608, 1978.

41. Larsen, V., Mogensen, B., Amris, C.J. and Storm, O.: Fibrinolytic enzyme in the treatment of patients with cancer. Danish Med Bull 11:137-140, 1964.

42. Elias, E.G. and Brugarolas, A.: The role of heparin in the chemotherapy of solid tumors: preliminary clinical trial in carcinoma of the lung. Cancer Chemother Rep 56:783-785, 1972.

43. Elias, E.G., Sepulveda, F. and Mink, I.: Increasing the efficiency of cancer chemotherapy with heparin: "clinical study." J Surg Oncol 5:189, 1973.

44. Elias, E.G., Shulka, S.K. and Mink, I.: Heparin and chemotherapy in the management of inoperable lung cancer. Cancer 36:129-136, 1975.

45. Edlis, H.E., Goudsmit, A., Brindley, C. and Niemetz, J.: Trial of heparin and cyclophosphamide (NSC-26271) in the treatment of lung cancer. Cancer Treat Rep 60:575-578, 1976.

46. Rohwedder, J.J. and Sagastume, E.: Heparin and polychemotherapy for treatment of lung cancer. Cancer Treat Rep 61: 1399-1401, 1977.

47. Elias, E.G., personal communication, 1979.

48. Stanford, C.F.: Anticoagulants in the treatment of small cell carcinoma of the bronchus. Thorax 34:113-116, 1979.

49. Salsali, M. and Cliffton, E.E. Superior vena caval obstruction with lung cancer. Ann Thoracic Surg 6:437-442, 1968.

50. Salsali, M. and Cliffton, E.E.: Superior vena caval obstruction in carcinoma of the lung. N Y St J Med 69:2875-2880, 1969.

51. Hoover, H.C., Jr., Ketcham, A.S., Millar, R.C. and Gralnick, H.R.: Osteosarcoma. Improved survival with anticoagulation and amputation. Cancer 41:2475-2480, 1978.

52. Thornes, R.D., Smyth, H., Browne, O. and Holland, P.D.J.: BCG plus protease 1 in malignant melanoma. Lancet 1:1386, 1973.

53. Williams, J.R.B. and Maugham, E.: Treatment of tumor metastases by defibrination. Br Med J 3:174, 1972.

54. Waddell, W.R.: Chemotherapy for carcinoma of the pancreas. Surg 74:420-429, 1973.

55. O'Halloran, M.J. and O'Meara, R.A.Q.: Clinical response in advanced breast cancer treated with protamine derivatives. Bull de la Soc Int de Chir 23:30-35, 1964.

56. Ries, J., Ludwig, H. and Appel, W.: Anticoagulants in the radiation treatment of carcinoma of the female genetalia. Med Welt 38:2042-2047, 1968.

57. Astedt, B., Glifberg, I., Mattsson, W. and Trope, C.: Arrest of growth of ovarian tumor by tranexamic acid. J Am Med Assn 238:154-155, 1977.

58. Astedt, B., Mattsson, W. and Trope, C.: Treatment of advanced breast cancer with chemotherapeutics and inhibition of coagulation and fibrinolysis. Acta Med Scand 201:491-493, 1977.

59. Kirsch, W.M., Van Buskirk, J.J., Schulz, D.W., and Tabuchi, K.: The biologic basis of malignant brain tumor therapy. Adv Neurol 15:301-313, 1976.

60. White, H. and Griffiths, J.D.: Circulating malignant cells and fibrinolysis during resection of colorectal cancer. Proc Roy Soc Med 69:467-469, 1976.

61. Thornes, R.D., Deasy, P.F., Carrol, R., Reen, D.J. and MacDonnell, J.D.: The use of the proteolytic enzyme Brinase to produce autocytotoxicity in patients with acute leukaemia and its possible role in immunotherapy. Cancer Res 32: 280-284, 1972.

62. Thornes, R.D.: Inhibition of antiplasmin, and effect of protease I in patients with leukemia. Lancet 2:1220-1223, 1968.

63. Thornes, R.D.: Fibrinolytic therapy of leukemia. J Roy Coll Surg Ireland 6:123-128, 1971.

64. Thornes, R.D., Smyth, H., Browne, O., O'Gorman, M., Reen, D.J., Farrell, D. and Holland, P.D.J.: The effects of proteolysis on the human immune mechanism in cancer. J Med 5:92-97, 1974.

65. Drapkin, R.L., Gee, T.S., Dowling, M.D., Arlin, Z., McKenzie, S., Kempin, S. and Clarkson, B.: Prophylactic heparin therapy in acute promyelocytic leukemia. Cancer 41: 2484-2490, 1978.

66. Nilsson, I.M., Bjorkman, S.E. and Andersson, L.: Clinical experiences with ε-aminocaproic acid (ε-ACA) as an anti-fibrinolytic agent. Acta Med Scand 170:487-509, 1961.

67. Gastpar, H.: Stickiness of platelets and tumor cells influenced by drugs, in Hematologic Reviews, Ambrus, J.L. (ed.), Marcel Dekker, Inc., 1972, pp. 1.

68. Ketcham, A.S., Sugarbaker, E.V., Ryan, J.J. and Orme, S.K.: Clotting factors and metastasis formation. Am J Roent III: 42-47, 1971.

69. Laki, K. and Yancey, S.T.: Fibrinogen and the tumor problem, in Fibrinogen, Laki, K. (ed.), Marcel Dekker, Inc., 1968, pp. 359.

70. Olwin, J.H.: Tumor metastasis and anticoagulants. Surg Gyn Obstet 132:1064-1066, 1971.

71. Wood, S., Jr.: Mechanism of establishment of tumor metastases, in Pathobiology Annual, Ioachim, H.L. (ed.), 1971, pp. 281.

72. Hilgard, P. and Thornes, R.D.: Anticoagulants in the treatment of cancer. Europ J Cancer 12: 755-762, 1976.

73. Zacharski, L.R., Henderson, W.G., Rickles, F.R., Forman, W.B., Cornell, C.J., Jr., Forcier, R.J., Harrower, H.H. and Johnson, R.D.: Rationale and experimental design for the VA Cooperative Study of anticoagulation (warfarin) in the treatment of cancer. Cancer 44:732-741, 1979.

74. Abercrombie, M.: The locomotory behavior of cells, *in* Cells and Tissues in Culture. Methods, Biology and Physiol 1, pp. 177-202, Academic Press, NY, 1965.

75. Zacharski, L.R. and Rosenstein, R.: Reduction of salivary tissue factor (TF) by warfarin therapy. Blood 53:366-374, 1979.

76. Chang, J.D. and Hill, T.C.: *In vitro* effect of sodium warfarin on DNA and RNA synthesis in mouse L1210 leukemia cells and Walker tumor cells. Oncology 28:332, 1973.

77. Kirsch, W.M., Schulz, D., Van Buskirk, J.J. and Young, E.E.: Effects of sodium warfarin and other carcinostatic agents on malignant cells: a study of drug synergy. J Med 5:69-82, 1974.

78. Jansen, C.R., Cronkite, E.P., Mather, G.C., Nielsen, N.O., Rai, K., Adamik, E.R. and Sipe, C.R.: Studies on lymphocytosis. II, The production of lymphocytosis by intravenous heparin in calves. Blood 20:443, 1962.

79. Kiricuta, I., Todorutin, C., Muresian, T. and Risca, R.: Prophylaxis of metastasis formation by unspecific immunologic stimulation associated with heparin therapy. Cancer 31:1392-1346, 1973.

80. Agostino, D. and Cliffton, E.E.: Decrease in pulmonary metastases: potentiation of nitrogen mustard effect by heparin and fibrinolysin. Ann Surg 157:400, 1963.

81. Hoover, H.C. and Ketcham, A.S.: Decreasing experimental metastasis formation with anticoagulation and chemotherapy. Surg Forum 26:173-174, 1975.

82. Ryan, J.J., Ketcham, A.S. and Wexler, H.: Warfarin treatment of mice bearing autochthonous tumors: effect on spontaneous metastases. Sci 162:1493-1494, 1968.

83. Hagmar, B.: Cell surface change and metastasis formation. A study on the effects of dextrans and heparin on tumor cells and experimental metastases in a syngeneic murine system. Acta Path Microbiol Scand 80:357-366, 1972.

84. Kohga, S.: Thromboplastic and fibrinolytic activities of ascites tumor cells in rats, with reference to their role in metastasis formation. Gann 69:461-170, 1978.

85. Fidler, I.J.: Tumor heterogeneity and the biology of cancer invasion and metastasis. Cancer Res 38:2651-1660, 1978.

86. De Vita, V.T., Jr.: The evolution of theropeutic research in cancer. N Eng J Med 298:907-910, 1978.

Malignancy and the Hemostatic System,
edited by M. B. Donati et al.
Raven Press, New York © 1981.

Haemostasis and Malignancy

J. F. Davidson and I. D. Walker

Royal Infirmary, Glasgow, United Kingdom

INTRODUCTION

In this Symposium the inter–relationships between haemostasis and malignancy have been explored in the light of current knowledge. Although there is much conflicting experimental evidence and whilst much of the work has been carried out in animal models and in tissue culture, certain trends have emerged which have relevance for future work in this field. There are clear and important interactions between platelets and malignant cells. Malignant disease has long been known to be associated with a high incidence of thrombosis and recently the importance of fibrinolysis in relation to cancer has been accepted. It is hoped that these advances in the basic science of malignancy will soon have clear implications for future developments in therapy.

PLATELETS AND MALIGNANCY

Malignant tissue has been shown to produce a platelet aggregating material which appears to be of a particulate nature and which seems to operate through the platelet release mechanism. Platelet aggregates can therefore be formed readily in relation to malignant tumours and these aggregates can provide a vehicle for the transport and dissemination of tumour cells. In certain animal models it has been shown that, if thrombocytopenia is induced, metastasis formation is reduced. Activated platelets release prostaglandins and other factors including growth factors and mitogenic factors which may contribute to the control of tumour growth.

It therefore seems logical to expect that inhibition of platelet function would have a beneficial effect on tumour growth and dissemination. To date trials of antiplatelet agents in malignant

disease have been rather disappointing, although not universally
so.

COAGULATION AND MALIGNANCY

Malignant tissue can promote activation of coagulation either by
its tissue thromboplastin or through a procoagulant which
activates FX directly.   In this way there is a tendency for fibrin
deposition to occur both in relation to the tumour and also at
distant sites in the vascular system.   Deposition of fibrin in the
periphery of the tumour probably protects the tumour against the
host's defence mechanisms and at the same time provides an
important lattice work for tumour spread.

Measures to reduce fibrin deposition would seem a potentially
promising means of controlling tumour growth and anticoagulant
therapy with Warfarin and other anticoagulants has been tried in
several clinical studies.   Predictably however, the results are
conflicting although certain authors do report evidence of clinical
benefit.   Coumarins appear to be the most promising in this
respect and interestingly their beneficial effect appears to be
independent of their anticoagulant effect.   It seems that their
anti-vitamin K action is more important and it may be that their
interference with vitamin K cellular physiology has a clinically
favourable effect in controlling malignant disease.   More clinical
studies of Coumarin as an adjunct to cancer chemotherapy
certainly seem justified.

FIBRINOLYSIS AND MALIGNANCY

Malignant tissue has been known for some time to be rich in
fibrinolytic activity.   This observation has recently been supported by experimental work with tissue culture, where malignant
cells in culture have been shown to produce a plasmin-like enzyme
and a plasminogen activator, which is similar or identical to
urokinase.   In addition, it has been shown that cells in culture,
when transformed by oncogenic viruses, produce abundant amounts
of plasminogen activator.   This viral induction of malignant
transformation appears to have the ability to "switch on" plasminogen activator production.

The significance of this tumour fibrinolytic activity has been the
subject of much study.   It has not been found to be correlated
with the degree of malignancy but nevertheless it has been
considered as a possible biological marker for neoplasia.

A radioimmune assay has been developed for this purpose and it remains to be seen if the early promise of this approach is substantiated.

Why do tumours generate fibrinolytic activator in such quantities? Is it merely a reflection of the cellular derangement of neoplasia or is it of biological importance to the tumour? As already discussed, the presence of fibrin appears to be advantageous to tumour growth and spread. On this principle increased fibrinolysis would seem likely to prove disadvantageous to the tumour. However,animal experiments have shown that pharmacological suppression of the increased fibrinolytic activity does not seem to advantage the tumour but rather appears to be clinically beneficial. The function of tumour plasminogen activator, therefore, remains something of a paradox.

CONCLUSION

Haemostasis appears quite clearly to have a significant role to play in malignant disease. Much experimental work is being devoted to this fascinating area at present and much of the new data is recorded in this volume. It is to be hoped, that as a result, therapeutic manipulation of the haemostatic mechanism may become a useful adjunct to cancer therapy.

Subject Index

A

Adenocarcinoma cells of, 9
    factor X and, 68
Adriamycin, 110
Ancrod treatment, 103
Anemia, microangiopathic
    hemolytic, 90
Angiotensin metabolism, 14–15
Anticoagulants, 103–127
    antimetastatic properties of, 103
    beneficial effects of, 59
    carefully controlled trials of, 120
    chemotherapy and, 57, 115–118
    complications in, 60
    immunotherapy and, 109–110
    local enivronment of cell and, 119–
      120
    maximal antimetastatic effect and,
      104
    mechanisms of, 119
    metastasis and, 60
    neoplastic cell and, 60
    poorly controlled studies on, 119
    pre-operative and post-operative,
      60
    previous treatment with, 114
    radiotherapy and, 109
    short-term vs long-term, 60
    time of administration of, 106
Antifibrinolytic agents, 119–120
Antiinflammatory agents,
    non-steroidal, 94
Antiplatelet drugs
    antimetastatic effects of, 104
    chemotherapy and, 57

B

Batroxobin, 94, 95
    antimetastatic effects of, 103

Bloodstream and metastasis, 5, 6
Breast cancer
    anticoagulation in, 117–118
    chemotherapy and anticoagulation
      in, 115
Bronchogenic malignancy, 9

C

Cancer cells. *See also* Tumors.
    blood clotting initiation by, 65–81
    circulating, wastage of, 12
    embolus of
      necrosis in, 8
      size of, 8
      types of, 13
      variations in components of, 13
    fibrin and, 57, 89
    interaction of endothelium and, 13
    motility of, warfarin and, 104
    movement into vascular lumen of,
      5
    organ retention of, microinjury
      hypothesis in, 15–22
    platelets and, 58
    preferential vessels for migration
      of, 5
    procoagulant activity of, 57–64,
      67–68
    prostacyclin generation by, 95
    size of, 9
    vessel wall penetration of, 7–8
Cancer cell–endothelial reactions,
    5–25
Cancer coagulant factor, 57
    physico-chemical properties of, 67
Cancer procoagulant A, 68–69
Central nervous system tumors, 118
Cervical carcinoma, 117

Chemotherapy and anticoagulation, 57, 115–118
Circulatory systems in tumor and host, 11
Clot deposition mechanism, 113–114
Coagulation
  hereditary disorders of, cancer incidence in, 114
  intravascular
    APL and, 58
    disseminated, 65, 113
    3LL tumor and, 90–91
  malignancy and, 130
  malignant tumors and, 57
  mechanism of
    activation in, 113
    malignancy and, 66
Colon carcinoma, 118
Complement and tumor vesicle binding, 28–29, 32
Coumadin, 60. *See also* Warfarin.
Coumarin
  antimetastatic effects of, 104
  cytotoxic drugs and, 109
  cytotoxic effects of, 104
  effects of, 95
  macrophage activation and, 107–108
  period of administration of, 94

D
Defibrination in disseminated malignant diseases, 1
Disseminated intravascular coagulation, 113
  incidence of, 65
  malignant disease and, 65

E
Endothelial cells
  cancer cell interaction with, 13
  injury to, 16
  plasminogen activator and, 14

prostaglandin and angiotensin metabolism by, 14–15
Epidermoid carcinoma, 9

F
Factor X activating activity, 58, 68–71
  cellular pathway of, 71
  direct and factor VII mediation of, 69–70
  malignant cell derivation of, 70–71
  mucus-producing adenocarcinomas and, 68
  phenprocoumon and, 107–109
  plasma recalcification time and, 69
  serine protease and, 71
  warfarin and, 96
Factor Xa generation, 69
Fibrin
  cancer cells and, 57
  cancer cell growth and, 89
  cancer cell invasion and, 66
  deposition of, 130
  formation of, host's contribution to, 66–67
  platelets and, metastasis and, 1
  tumor deposition of, 93
Fibrinogen turnover, 65–66
Fibrinolysis, 130–131
Fibrinolytic therapy, 115

H
Hemostatic system
  abnormal, 65
  metastasis and, 2
  pharmacologic modulation of, 92–96
  primary tumor and, 91
Heparin
  antimetastatic effects of, 103
  leukemia and, 59
  lung cancer and, 61, 115–116
Historical aspects of coagulation in malignancy, 113

Hodgkin's disease, 115
Host, circulatory systems of tumor
    and, 11

I
Immunotherapy and anticoagulants,
    109–110
Intravasation process, 8

L
Leucocyte procoagulant activity, 72
Leukemia
    acute lymphoblastic, fibrinolytic
        activity in, 59
    acute myelogenous, fibrinolytic
        activity in, 59
    chronic myeloid, anticoagulation
        and chemotherapy in, 115
    fibrinolytic agent in, 59, 118
    hemorrhagic syndrome in, 59
    hypergranular promyelocytic
        heparin treatment in, 59
    intravascular coagulation in, 58
Lung cancer
    anticoagulation and chemotherapy
        in, 115–116
    heparin and, 61

M
Macrophage activation, 107–108
Malignancy. *See also* Cancer cells;
    Tumors.
    genetic variation in, 1
    action of tumor inducing agents in,
        1
    probability of chromosomal lesion
        in, 2
    metastatic. *See* Metastasis.
Melanoma, malignant, 116–117
Metastasis
    anticoagulation therapy and, 60
    bloodstream in, 5, 6
    cell clumps vs single cells in, 9
    coumadin and, 60

drug effects on, 93
fibrin and, 66
fibrin and platelets in, 1
haemostatic process in, 2
microinjury hypothesis in, 15–22
pharmacology in, 94
physiological factors in, 2
prevention of, 22
warfarin and, 60
Microangiopathy, 91
Microcirculatory units, 15
Microinjury hypothesis, 15–22
    cell size in, 20
    endothelial injury in, 16
    fate of tumor cells in, 21
    island-forming tumor strains in, 21
    ready cancer cell attachment in, 15
    shedding characteristics in, 21
    single cell strains in, 21
    site of injury in, 20
    tumor cell showers in, 18
    unplugging system in, 20–21
Migration pore, 8

N
Necrosis and cancer cell embolus, 8
Neovascularization, 66

O
Osteogenic sarcoma, 116
Ovary, papillary adenocarcinoma of,
    117

P
Pharmacology. *See also*
    Anticoagulants; *individual*
    drugs.
    artificial and spontaneous lung
        metastases and, 93
    batroxobin and, 95
    coumarin derivatives and, 95
    hemostatic system and, 92–96
    length of treatment with, 94

Pharmacology *(contd.)*
  non-steroidal antiinflammatory
    agents and, 94
  periods of administration with, 94
  platelet aggregation inhibitors in,
    94
  prostacyclin inhibition by, 95
  prostaglandin inhibition by, 94–95
  snake venom enzymes and, 95
Phenprocoumon
  antimetastatic effects of, 103
  cytotoxic effects of, 104
  factor X activating activity and,
    107–109
  length of treatment with, 94
  long-term therapy with, 104–105
Plasminogen activator, 83–88
  action of, 14
  malignant ovarian tissue and, 83
  normal ovarian tissue and, 83
  urokinase and, 83–85
    antiserum, 84
    labelled, 84
    ovarian carcinoma blood and,
      85
    ovarian tumors and, 85–87
    peripheral blood and, 85–87
    purification of, 83–84
    radioimmunoassay for, 84–85,
      87
    uterine cavity wash and, 85–87
Plasma and tumor vesicle binding, 28
Plasma prothrombin complex
    activity, 96
Plasma recalcification time, 69
Platelets
  cancer cells and, 58
  increased turnover of, 65–66
  malignancy and, 129–130
  pseudopodia production by, 9
  vessel wall aggregation of, 8
  washed, platelet aggregating
    material and, 50–51
Platelet aggregation inhibitors, 94

Platelet aggregating material, 37–55
  activities or sites of, 52
  boiling and, 46–47
  cell culture for, 38
  cell extracts and, 51
  cell plasma membrane
    component and, 53
  centrifugation of, 40, 47
  chemical constituents and physical
    nature of, 53
  chemicals, enzymes, reagents and,
    42–43
  collagen and, 53
  destruction of, 52
  enzymes and, 41, 46–47
  extraction of, 38–39
  free fatty acids and, 52
  heat factor for, 52
  in vitro measurement of, 39–40
  inhibitors of, 43–44, 52
  lipid analysis of, 40–41, 47–48
  lipid moiety and, 52
  mechanism of action of, 52
  non-inhibition of, 44–45
  non-ionic detergents and, 46–47
  normal cells and, 51
  phospholipids and, 53
  preparation of PRP and PPP for,
    39
  preparation of washed human
    platelets for, 39
  protease inhibitors and, 45
  serotonin release and, 41–42, 44
  sialic acid and, 53
  sonification and, 46–47
  synergism between epinephrine
    and, 50
  thrombofax and, 52–53
  tumor lines in, 9–10
  tumor vesicles in, 27–35
    action of, 28
    cofactor activity in, 33
    complement in, 28–29, 32
    C3-deficient rat PRP in, 32

fraction concentration in, 28
genetically C4-deficient guinea
    pig sera in, 31
heat-treated rat plasma in, 31
heparinized rat plasma in, 30
radioactive studies in, 30
role of plasma in, 28
thrombin in, 33–34
vesicle binding in, 28
vesicle preparation and, 27–28
vitamine-K dependent plasma
    protein in, 32–33
as type III tumor cells, 52
urea extract and, 43
viral transformants and, 51
washed platelets and, 50–51
whole cells in, 43
Procoagulant activity of cancer cell,
    57–64, 67–68
enzymatic action of, 57–58
intravascular coagulation and, 58
leucocytes and, 72
pathophysiological, 72–73
physico-chemical properties of, 67
rich sources of, 57
thromboplastic, 67–68
tissue factor definition in, 57–58
transglutaminase activities and, 58
tumor variation and, 67
warfarin and, 96
Procoagulant research
allogenic tumors in, 89
dead cells or inert material
    injection in, 90
i.v. injection of cancer cells in, 89–
    90
Lewis Lung Carcinoma cell
    injection in, 90
Walker 256 Carcinosarcoma
    injection in, 90
Promyelocytes and tissue factor
    activity, 59, 72
Prostacyclin generation, 95
Prostaglandin

drug inhibition of, 94–95
endothelial metabolism of, 14–15
Pseudopodia, platelet, 9

R
Radiotherapy and anticoagulants,
    109

S
Shedding characteristics, 11
microinjury hypothesis and, 21
Snake venom enzymes, 95

T
Thrombin and platelet aggregation,
    33–34
Thromboembolic events, 113
Thromboplastic activity, 67–68
qualitative differences in, 68
quantitative differences in, 68
Thromboplastin, tissue, 114
Thrombosis and cancer surgery, 65
Tissue factor activity, 72–73, 114
leukemic promyelocytes and, 72
Transglutaminase activities, 58
Tumors. *See also* Cancer cells.
allogenic, 89
central nervous system, 118
circulatory systems of host and, 11
fibrin deposition and, 93
neovascularization of, 66
primary
    hemostatic system and, 91
    metastatic nodules and, 91
    microangiopathy and, 91
3LL
    characteristics and coagulation
        changes of, 91–92
    intravascular coagulation and,
        90–91
Tumor angiogenesis factor, 2–3
Tumor vesicles. *See also* Platelet
    aggreation, tumor vesicles in.

Tumor vesicles *(contd.)*
  binding of
    complement in, 28–29, 32
    plasma in, 28

U
Urokinase
  molecular, 87
  plasminogen activator and, 83–85

V
Vascular lumen and cancer cell
    movement, 5
Vena cava malignant obstruction,
  116
Vessel wall
  migration pore on, 8
  platelet aggregates on, 8
Vitamin K, 130
  deficiency of, 106–107

W
Walker 256 Carcinosarcoma, 90
Warfarin
  adriamycin and, 110
  antimetastatic effects of, 95, 103
  cancer cell motility and, 104
  factor X activating activity and, 96
  high doses of, 104
  human clinical trials with, 115
  length of treatment with, 94
  low concentrations of, 104
  lung tumor deposits and, 106
  macrophage inhibitors and, 107
  metastasis and, 60
  osteogenic sarcoma and, 116
  period of action of, 106
  plasma prothrombin complex
    activity and, 96
  procoagulant activity and, 96
  short-term, 104
  radiotherapy and, 109
  vitamin K-dependent proteins and,
    95–96